Dedication

To Drew and Ty for their patience and boundless energy.

Single
Best
Questions

Psychiatry Book 2 – 2004

ANSWER SHEET

There are 250 blocks below to record your answers.

1	26	51	76	101	126	151	176	201	226
2	27	52	77	102	127	152	177	202	227
3	28	53	78	103	128	153	178	203	228
4	29	54	79	104	129	154	179	204	229
5	30	55	80	105	130	155	180	205	230
6	31	56	81	106	131	156	181	206	231
7	32	57	82	107	132	157	182	207	232
8	33	58	83	108	133	158	183	208	233
9	34	59	84	109	134	159	184	209	234
10	35	60	85	110	135	160	185	210	235
11	36	61	86	111	136	161	186	211	236
12	37	62	87	112	137	162	187	212	237
13	38	63	88	113	138	163	188	213	238
14	39	64	89	114	139	164	189	214	239
15	40	65	90	115	140	165	190	215	240
16	41	66	91	116	141	166	191	216	241
17	42	67	92	117	142	167	192	217	242
18	43	68	93	118	143	168	193	218	243
19	44	69	94	119	144	169	194	219	244
20	45	70	95	120	145	170	195	220	245
21	46	71	96	121	146	171	196	221	246
22	47	72	97	122	147	172	197	222	247
23	48	73	98	123	148	173	198	223	248
24	49	74	99	124	149	174	199	224	249
25	50	75	100	125	150	175	200	225	250

Please remove from the book before beginning.

1. The hallmark feature of social phobia that distinguishes it from agoraphobia is:

   A) Social phobia may occur with or without panic disorder, while agoraphobia only occurs in conjunction with panic disorder
   B) Social phobia describes the fear of embarrassing oneself in social situations, while agoraphobia describes the fear of being unable to escape during a panic attack
   C) Social phobics only fear people, while agoraphobics fear people and places
   D) Social phobia is often alleviated by the presence of a companion, while agoraphobia is exacerbated by it
   E) Social phobics respond best to a combination of pharmacotherapy and behavioral approaches, while agoraphobics are best treated with behavioral techniques alone

2. A 32-year-old Malaysian male, recent immigrant to the United States was brought to the ER by police for erratic public behavior. According to the police report, the man was running around in circles, shouting incomprehensible phrases at the top of his lungs, and provoking fights with strangers on the street.

   Leading diagnostic possibilities include all of the following **EXCEPT**?

   A) A Culture Bound Syndrome
   B) Cocaine intoxication
   C) Malingering
   D) Obsessive Compulsive Disorder
   E) Schizophrenia

3. Which one of the following is a common, cardinal feature of narcolepsy?

   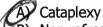
   A) Cataplexy
   B) Non refreshing sleep attacks
   C) Increased rate of job related accidents
   D) Sleep paralysis
   E) Response to stimulants

4.   A 67-year-old male with a 10-year history of multiple myeloma commits suicide by hanging himself with a rope.

Which of the following statements about the patient is **FALSE**?

A) He likely suffers from an underlying psychiatric illness
B) He may have decreased levels of 5-hydroxyindoleactic acid in his cerebrospinal fluid
C) His diagnosis of multiple myeloma heightened his risk of suicide
D) He likely saw his physician in the 6 months prior to his suicide
E) His age put him at an increased risk for attempting suicide compared with those younger than him

5.   A 25-year-old college student wrecked her car while driving at high speeds on the highway at 3 AM. In the Emergency Room (ER), while being treated for minor lacerations, she started to run naked through the hallway. She was psychomotorically agitated and her affect was expansive. Her friends report that she has been acting "strangely" for over a week, including not sleeping and not eating. When the psychiatrist interviewed her in the ER, she reported hearing voices telling her that she is a bad person and that she should kill herself.

Given the above description, the **MOST** likely diagnosis is:

A) Bipolar I, most recent episode depressed, with mood incongruent hallucinations and delusions
B) Bipolar I, most recent episode depressed, with mood congruent hallucinations and delusions
C) Bipolar I, most recent episode manic, with mood congruent hallucinations and delusions
D) Bipolar I, most recent episode manic, with mood incongruent hallucinations and delusions
E) Bipolar I, most recent episode mixed, with mood incongruent hallucinations and delusions

6.   Relative to haloperidol, olanzapine is **MORE** likely to:

A) Cause constipation
B) Induce a major increase in a patient's weight
C) Precipitate akinesia in a patient with Parkinson's disease
D) Lead to an acute dystonia
E) Prolong the QT interval on EKG (electrocardiogram)

7. A 48-year-old male auto mechanic complains of chronic, non-restorative sleep, frequent awakenings, daytime fatigue and poor concentration. He estimates that he sleeps about 5 out of the 9 hours he spends in bed. His only medication is ibuprofen for chronic lower back pain.

    On exam, he is 40 pounds above his ideal body weight and he has mildly elevated blood pressure.

    Which one of the following is **LEAST** useful in further evaluating the patient's sleep/wake complaints?

    A) Polysomnography
    B) Tape recording of respiratory sounds during sleep
    C) Head CT without contrast
    D) Beck Depression Inventory
    E) Interview with bed partners

8. A key component of cognitive-behavioral therapy for panic disorder is "interoceptive exposures."

    This technique is **BEST** described by which of the following?

    A) Exposing the patient to difficult emotional material from childhood to uncover unconscious fears and motivations
    B) Exposing the patient to cognitive misinterpretations of somatic sensations using thought records and cognitive rehearsals
    C) Exposing the patient to scenarios that evoke anxiety and panic using guided imagery
    D) Exposing the patient to imagery and body sensations that evoke anxiety while the patient performs rapid tracking eye movements
    E) Exposing the patient to panic like somatic sensations by recreating the sensations during the session

Medtext Medical World, Inc.

9. A 33-year-old woman G2P1 in her 24th week of pregnancy was brought to the ER by her husband for treatment of a burn to her hand. Over the last 3 days she has become preoccupied with demons and has been lighting candles in every room of the house to keep the evil spirits away. By the husband's report, the patient has not slept in 5 nights because she has been up late doing "Internet research" for a new book she is writing on exorcism.

On exam she is psychomotorically agitated and her mood is dysphoric.

The patient has a history of bipolar disorder and has been on 900 mg of lithium carbonate for the past 5 years. She has continued to take the medication during her pregnancy.

Which of the following statements regarding the treatment of this patient is **MOST** accurate?

    A) Lithium is the best treatment for the patient since she may be having a mixed episode

    B) This patient's lithium dose should be decreased by half a couple of weeks prior to delivery

    C) The patient should have been switched to valproic acid at the start of pregnancy to decrease the risk of teratogenicity   NO

    D) The safest intervention now is to stop all medications and hospitalize the patient

    E) This patient could currently benefit from antipsychotics but the risk of teratogenicity far outweighs the benefits

10.   A 52-year-old female is brought to the ER by her concerned husband of 25 years. He states that his wife has been acting very strangely of late and spends many hours a day monitoring the activities of the neighbors. She is concerned that the neighbors are "spying on her for the FBI." For the last month, she has been convinced that they have bugged the vents in her home so they can listen to her every move." She hears them whispering all day long about how they are going to kill her. This morning she noticed a cut on her forehead and accused the neighbors of implanting a transmitter in her brain while she slept. The husband states that his wife was her normal self until 4 months ago when she started to become hypervigilant. Recently, she has become so preoccupied that she is unable to work or do her usual household chores.

Regarding this patient's diagnosis, which one of the following statements is **MOST** accurate?

A) A significant history of depression coexisting with the above symptoms would preclude a diagnosis of schizophrenia
B) This patient's age would rule out a diagnosis of schizophrenia
C) The duration of this patient's symptoms is consistent with a diagnosis of schizophrenia
D) The degree of functional impairment seen in this patient suggests a diagnosis of schizophrenia over a diagnosis of a mood disorder
E) The content of this patient's delusions suggests a diagnosis of major depressive disorder with psychotic features over a diagnosis of schizophrenia

(11-15)

A 70-year-old male with a known history of chronic atrial fibrillation was well when he retired to bed. He was found by his wife 2 hours later, unable to move his right side, unable to speak and with eyes deviated to the left.

11.   Based on this history the **LEAST** likely diagnosis is:

A) Carotid dissection
B) Embolic stroke
C) Hemorrhage in a tumor
D) Todd palsy
E) Brainstem stroke below the pons

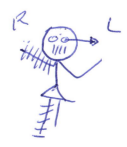

                    Medtext Medical World, Inc.

12. Initial CT scan discloses no abnormality.

The initial **FIRST** step in management is:

A) Intravenous rt-PA ✓
B) Intra-arterial rt-PA
C) Intravenous low molecular weight heparin
D) Warfarin (Coumadin)
E) None of the above

13. The ED physician decides to administer rt-PA:

A) You would consider it appropriate therapy ✓
B) You would advice him to consider intra-arterial rt-PA
C) You would advise him to obtain a surgical consultation
D) Advise anticonvulsants
E) Advise gradual warfarin (Coumadin) after 2-3 weeks

14. The patient shows gradual worsening of his sensorium.

All are true **EXCEPT**:

A) This may be natural consequence of his stroke
B) This may be due to secondary bleeding
C) Patient may be in non-convulsive status
D) Metabolic derangements may explain the worsening sensorium
E) Subarachnoid hemorrhage has occurred as a consequence of his stroke

15. Carotid studies reveal a 99% stenosis of the left internal carotid artery.

Appropriate management would be:

A) Delayed surgery ✓
B) Immediate CEA
C) Lifelong anticoagulation with warfarin (Coumadin)
D) Lifelong anticoagulation with heparin
E) Hemispherectomy

Medtext Medical World, Inc.

(16-20)

Lateral Medullary infarct

A 77-year-old male was seen because of acute onset of vertigo, vomiting and dysarthria, dysphagia. → *diff. swallowing*

16.   All the following are important differential diagnosis **EXCEPT**:

   A) Lateral medullary syndrome
   B) Anterior cerebellar artery occlusion
   C) Internal carotid artery occlusion
   D) Basilar thrombosis
   E) Medial medullary syndrome

speech impairment

movement vol of the palate voluntary → NO

17.   MRI of the brain reveals a diffusion weighted (DWI) hyperintensity in the lateral medullary region and multiple DWI negative white matter lesions

   The patient **MOST** likely had

   A) A single acute infarct in the lateral medullary region
   B) Multiple acute infarcts
   C) Hemorrhage in the medulla
   D) Venous thrombosis
   E) None of the above

18.   Lateral medullary infarcts are characterized by all the following **EXCEPT**:

   A) Dysphagia
   B) Dysarthria
   C) Hemiparesis *No*
   D) Facial loss of pain and temperature
   E) Nystagmus

19.   Prognosis for recovery is usually:

        A) Poor
        B) Guarded
        C) Excellent
        D) Not known
        E) Depends on the individual patient

20.   The **MOST** debilitating symptom of this syndrome is:

        A) Dysphagia
        B) Dysarthria
        C) Seizures
        D) Hemiparesis
        E) Diplopia

(21-25)

A patient is seen in the sleep clinic with complaints of violent behavior at night with injuries to his spouse. The patient recalls some of that behavior.

21.   The **MOST** likely diagnosis would be:

        A) Seizures
        B) Malingering
        C) REM behavior disorder
        D) Cataplexy
        E) Drug withdrawal

22.   If he had seizures, the **LEAST** likely diagnosis would be:

        A) Complex partial seizures
        B) Frontal lobe cingulate seizures
        C) Rolandic epilepsy
        D) Opercular seizures
        E) All of the above

23.   EEG during a seizure is **MOST** likely to be normal in:

A) Frontal lobe epilepsy
B) Complex partial seizures
C) Generalized seizures
D) All of the above
E) None of the above.

24.   The **MOST** appropriate initial investigation for this patient would be:

A) Polysomnography
B) Depth recorded EEG
C) Surface EEG
D) Visual evoked potentials
E) All of the above

25.   REM behavior disorder is **BEST** treated by:

A) Phenytoin (Dilantin)
B) Barbiturates
C) SSRI
D) Clonazepam (Klonapin)
E) Acupuncture

(26-30)

A 47-year-old woman presented with vertical diplopia of acute onset. This was the only symptom. The neurological examination revealed a third nerve paresis. Pupillary reflexes were normal.

26.   The **MOST** likely anatomical localization of this patient's deficit is:

A) Orbit
B) 3rd Nerve (fascicular)
C) Midbrain
D) Cortex
E) Pons

Medtext Medical World, Inc.

27. Given the presentation, the **MOST** likely etiology of this lesion is

   A) Compression of the midbrain
   B) Tentorial herniation
   C) Cavernous sinus thrombosis
   D) Ischemic neuropathy
   E) Pontine hemorrhage

28. The following would be appropriate in investigating this problem except

   A) MRI of the brain
   B) Fasting Blood Sugar
   C) Vasculitic work-up
   D) Chest CT scan
   E) ESR

29. Prognosis for recovery in this case is:

   A) Poor
   B) Good
   C) Delayed, with near complete recovery
   D) Delayed with little recovery
   E) All of the above

30. In a well controlled diabetic, risk of recurrence is:

   A) Low
   B) Moderate
   C) High
   D) Independent of the diabetic status
   E) All of the above

(31-35)

Restless Leg syndrome

AJ is a 40-year-old male who is seen because of excessive daytime sleepiness. He has noticed an ill described feeling of discomfort in his legs especially in the evenings. He lives alone.

31.   The **MOST** appropriate initial step is:

   A) Detailed history and examination ✓
   B) MRI
   C) EEG
   D) CT scan
   E) Multiple sleep latency test (MSLT)

32.   His clinical examination may reveal:

   A) Loss of sensations in the legs with areflexia
   B) Resting tremors of the upper extremities
   C) No findings
   D) Conjunctival pallor
   E) All of the above are possibilities

33.   The **MOST** appropriate investigative step would be:

   A) Polysomnography
   B) Multiple sleep latency test
   C) EEG
   D) MRI
   E) Carotid Doppler studies

34.   The polysomnogram is **LIKELY** to reveal:

   A) Sleep fragmentation ✓
   B) Periodic leg movements of sleep ✓
   C) Obstructive apnea
   D) Cardiac arrhythmia
   E) A and B

Medtext Medical World, Inc.

35.   Additional abnormalities that might be seen **MOST** commonly:

Restless leg syndrome may be associated with Anemia, Iron deficiency

Tx → Sinemet - agonist, Dopamine - agonist or Klonopin, Neurontin + opioids

(A) Low serum ferritin
B) Low sodium
C) High osmolarity
D) Acanthocytosis
E) Low iron binding capacity

peripheral Neuropathy medication and EPS

early gait disturbance + incontinence - Headache + Dementia

(36-40)

NPH →

A 75-year-old Caucasian male was seen in the neurology clinic with a history of recent incontinence and headaches. Over the past 6 months he has developed a drunken gait with recurrent falls. He has stopped handling the household accounts because he makes frequent mistakes.

Brain Tumor

36.   The examination reveals papilledema without focal deficits and bilateral Babinski's.

These findings are **MOST** compatible with:

A) Alzheimer's disease
B) Mesial temporal sclerosis
(C) Midline brain tumor
D) CVA
E) Toxic encephalopathy

37.   In the absence of papilledema, all of the following features suggest NPH **EXCEPT**:

(A) Early dementia
B) Gait ataxia
C) Incontinence
D) Ventriculomegaly out of proportion to cortical atrophy on CT scans
E) All of the above

Medtext Medical World, Inc.

38.   Head CT may show all the following **EXCEPT**:

    A) Ventriculomegaly ✓
    B) Midline brain tumor ✓
    C) 4th ventricle tumor ✓
    D) Aqueductal stenosis ✓
    E) Cortical atrophy alone —→ *AZ or old age*

39.   The **MOST** predictive test of subsequent improvement of Normal Pressure Hydrocephalus (NPH) with a VP shunt is:

    A) CT scan
    B) MRI scan with gadolinium
    C) Clearance of Radioactive labeled tracers from the CSF
    D) Clinical response to removal of 30 cc of CSF ✓
    E) Psychometry

40.   A successful VP shunt is expected to help in all the following **EXCEPT**:

    A) Ventriculomegaly ✓
    B) Midline brain tumor ✓
    C) 4th ventricle tumor ✓
    D) Aqueductal stenosis ✓
    E) Cortical atrophy alone

Medtext Medical World, Inc.

(41-45)

A 44-year-old male woke up with loss of vision in both eyes. Three days prior to the onset of symptoms he had a severe pulsating headache with preceding blurred vision and numbness in the right arm. That lasted for 30 minutes. The weekend covering physician had prescribed Cafergot (2 tablets at onset and 1 every hour, maximum of 5/d. After 4 tablets his headache was completely relieved. When he went to bed the night before the onset of visual loss he was feeling normal. Neurological examination revealed bilateral central visual loss sparing the peripheral fields. The remaining neurological examination was normal.

41. From the history and examination the **MOST** likely site of the lesion is:

   A) Parietal
   B) Occipital involving area 18
   C) Occipital involving area 19
   D) Occipital involving the occipital pole in the dominant side
   E) Occipital involving bilateral occipital poles

42. Possible causes of loss of vision may include all of the following **EXCEPT**:

   A) Medications
   B) Complicated Migraine
   C) Tumors with raised intracranial pressure
   D) Multiple Sclerosis
   E) Retinitis pigmentosa

43. Causes of visual loss in patients with migraine are all the following **EXCEPT**:

   A) complicated migraine
   B) Ischemic stroke
   C) Medications
   D) Antiphospholipid antibody syndrome
   E) Multiple sclerosis

44. Contraindications to vasoconstrictors and Trip tans include all **EXCEPT**:

   A) Heart disease
   B) Hypertension
   C) Hemiplegic migraine
   D) Basilar migraine
   E) Migraine with aura

45. All are risk factors for stroke in patients presenting with headaches **EXCEPT**:

   A) Migraine with aura
   B) Antiphospholipid antibody syndrome
   C) Severe hypertension
   D) Anti- migraine medications
   E) Muscle contraction headaches

(46-50)

Anticardiolipin Antibody syndrome

AJ is an 18-year-old female who presented with a history of recurrent headaches. The headaches are unilateral and associated with nausea, photophobia and sonophobia with a frequency of 2 per month. There is no aura or focal neurological deficits associated with the headaches. About 2 years before the onset of these symptoms the patient was diagnosed with Immune Thrombocytopenic Purpura (ITP). However there were no antiplatelet antibodies evident. General physical and comprehensive neurological examinations were normal.

46. All the following are important in the initial work-up of this patient **EXCEPT**:

   A) MRI/ CT scan of the brain
   B) Serological tests for SLE
   C) Family history
   D) History of drug abuse
   E) Nerve conduction studies

*Unilateral Headache
Nausea – photophobia
and sonophobia*

Medtext Medical World, Inc.

47. The patients low platelet counts may be explained by all the following **EXCEPT**:

    A) ITP
    B) Infections associated with thrombocytopenia
    C) CADASIL
    D) SLE
    E) Antiphospholipid antibody syndrome

Cerebral Autosomal Dominant

48. The **MOST** likely diagnosis in this patient is:

    A) SLE
    B) Subdural hematoma
    C) Anticardiolipin antibody syndrome
    D) Brain tumor
    E) CADASIL

49. The **BEST** treatment for the patient is:

    A) Prophylactic treatment with antimigraine medications
    B) Low dose aspirin
    C) Warfarin (Coumadin)
    D) Neurosurgical intervention
    E) High dose oral steroids

50. The **BEST** treatment for this patient in pregnancy if the MRI reveals an ischemic infarct would be:

    A) Warfarin
    B) Aspirin
    C) Low dose steroids
    D) Heparin
    E) Stress reduction therapy

Medtext Medical World, Inc.

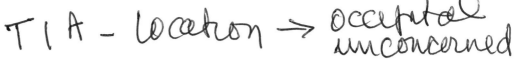

(51-55)

A 22-year-old male with no significant past medical history had a sudden transient onset of confusion while he was at work. He was unable to understand any commands, but appeared relatively unconcerned. The observers denied any history of unconsciousness, falls, weakness of one side of the body or problems with gait. His past medical history was significant for recurrent episodes of cyanosis and he seemed to find temporary relief with squatting. Otherwise he was a full term normal delivery although his physical development was slow.

Examination revealed that the patient was alert and did not obey verbal commands. His speech was fluent and sometimes difficult to understand. The remaining examination was normal. All his symptoms resolved within 30 minutes of onset.

51.   The **BEST** localization 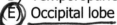 for this patient's symptoms is:

        A) Thalamus
        B) Pons
        C) Temporal lobe
        D) Temporoparietal lobes
        E) Occipital lobe

52.   All the following are relevant investigations **EXCEPT**:

        A) MRI scan of the brain with MR Angiography
        B) A full metabolic workup
        C) Drug and toxin screen
        D) Review past medical history of alcoholism
        E) Neuropsychiatric intervention

53.   The **MOST** likely diagnosis is:

        A) Seizures
        B) Stroke
        C) Drug intoxication
        D) Wernicke encephalopathy and psychosis
        E) Transient ischemic attack

Medtext Medical World, Inc.

54.   Appropriate management would be:

   A) Discharge home if the CT scan is normal and give instructions to take an aspirin, follow-up in the neurology clinic the next few days
   B) Admit for a detailed work-up
   C) Discharge home if the EEG was normal
   D) Discharge home if the Metabolic and toxic screen was normal
   E) Discharge home if the MRI was normal

55.   The prognosis of patients with a TIA discharged from the Emergency Department for outpatient follow-up is:

   A) Normal survival
   B) 20% develop a stroke within 2 days
   C) 5% develop a stroke within 2 days
   D) They are more likely to develop seizures
   E) None of the above

(56-61)   *Temporal Arteritis*

A 66-year-old female patient was admitted to the neurological services with acute loss of vision in the left eye and severe headache. The examination revealed reduced pulsations over the temporal arteries and swelling of the optic discs with hemorrhages.

56.   All the following are reasonable in the differential diagnosis **EXCEPT**:

        A) Stroke
        B) Temporal Arteritis
        C) Tumor with hemorrhage
        D) Sub arachnoid hemorrhage
        E) Migraine with aura

57.   The initial MRI scan of the brain with contrast was reported as normal.

        This reasonably excludes the diagnosis of which **ONE** of the following:

        A) Tumor
        B) Migraine
        C) Subarachnoid hemorrhage
        D) Temporal arteritis
        E) Stroke

58.   The **NEXT** step in management should be to perform:

        A) Lumbar puncture
        B) CBC, ESR, ANA, SACE
        C) Urgent brain biopsy
        D) Evoked potentials (visual and somatosensory)
        E) Neurophthalmic consult

Medtext Medical World, Inc.

59.   If the LP is negative, the **BEST** approach to initial treatment should be:

   A) Low dose aspirin
   B) Warfarin (Coumadin)
   C) Neurosurgical intervention if the LP is normal
   D) High dose steroids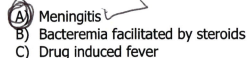
   E) Wait for a temporal artery biopsy before initiating steroids

60.   Soon after admission the patient developed high grade fever and started to lose vision in the other eye.

   Your **MAIN** concern at this stage will be that this patient has developed:

   A) Meningitis
   B) Bacteremia facilitated by steroids
   C) Drug induced fever
   D) Cavernous sinus thrombosis
   E) Sagittal sinus thrombosis

61.   A 32-year-old woman is terrified of dogs and refuses to leave her house to go to work because she may see a dog on the street.

   Diagnostic impression:

   A) Panic disorder with agoraphobia because she will not leave her home
   B) Malingering to avoid work
   C) Factitious disorder to avoid work
   D) Specific phobia because she is afraid of dogs
   E) Social phobia because she is afraid of work place

62. Before she can go to sleep at night, a 26-year-old woman counts the tiles on the ceiling at least five times. She has had a few minor car accidents because she has been distracted by counting traffic lights.

Diagnostic impression:

A) Obsessive compulsive disorder
B) Obsessive compulsive personality disorder
C) Schizotypal personality disorder
D) Schizophrenia
E) Cyclothymia

63. **True** of obsessive compulsive disorder:

A) More common in women than men *men = woman occurs in 2-3% population*
B) Occurs in less than 1% of population
C) Concordance rates are same for monozygotic and dizygotic twins *Mono > Dizy*
D) Obsessive Compulsive Disorder symptoms may first appear following a significant life stressor
E) Most patients have limited or no insight and unmotivated to eliminate the symptoms *insight present*

64. A 39-year-old woman says that she frequently experiences "palpitations," shortness of breath, and chronic indigestion. She says that for as long as she can remember, she has felt "tense and nervous." *GAD = Last at least 6 months 50% onset occur in childhood*

Diagnostic impression:

A) Panic disorder
B) Social phobia
C) Generalized anxiety disorder
D) Dependent personality
E) Dysthymia

65.   A 36-year-old woman who was raped 5 years ago has recurrent vivid memories of the rape accompanied by intense anxiety. These memories frequently intrude during her daily activities, and nightmares about the event often wake her. Her symptoms intensified when a coworker was raped 2 months ago.

Diagnostic impression:

A) Borderline personality disorder
B) Post traumatic stress disorder
C) Acute stress response
D) Dependent personality disorder
E) Adjustment disorder with mixed disturbance of mood and thought

66.   **True** of posttraumatic stress disorder (PTSD):

A) Lifetime prevalence of 15%
B) 75% of patients recover completely within 3 months
C) Group therapy should only be recommended if diagnosis confirmed
D) Psychopharmacologic intervention is contraindicated
E) Up to half of victims of catastrophic events will meet criteria for PTSD

67.   A 44-year-old woman has a 20-year history of vague and chronic physical complaints. She says that she has always been sick but that her doctors never seem to identify the problem and cannot help her.

Diagnostic impression:

A) Somatization disorder
B) Conversion disorder
C) Hypochondriasis
D) Factitious disorder
E) Body dysmorphic disorder

Medtext Medical World, Inc.

68. A 28-year-old woman experiences a sudden loss of vision, but appears unconcerned. She reports that just before the onset of her blindness, she saw her child dart into the street.

    Diagnostic impression:

    A) Conversion disorder
    B) Somatization disorder
    C) Hypochondriasis
    D) Factitious disorder
    E) Shared psychotic disorder

69. A 42-year-old man says that he has been "ill" for most of his life. He has seen many doctors but is angry with most of them because they ultimately referred him to mental health clinicians. He now fears that he has stomach cancer because his stomach makes noises after he eats. Many of his previous "illnesses" also seem to be amplified responses to normal physical sensations.

    Diagnostic impression:

    A) Somatization disorder
    B) Conversion disorder
    C) Factitious disorder
    D) Delusional disorder
    E) Hypochondriasis

70. A 28-year-old woman seeks blepharoplasty for her "sagging" eyelids. She rarely goes out in the daytime because she believes that this characteristic makes her look "like an old lady." On physical examination, her eyelids appear completely normal.

    Diagnostic impression:

    A) Somatoform disorder not otherwise specified
    B) Body dysmorphic disorder
    C) Factitious disorder
    D) Hypochondriasis
    E) Somatization disorder

Medtext Medical World, Inc.

71. A 40-year-old man who had a minor knee injury playing ball 11 months ago continues to complain of severe knee pain, although there is little or no evidence of any abnormality.

Diagnostic impression:

A) Conversion disorder
B) Pain disorder
C) Hypochondriasis
D) Factitious disorder
E) Adjustment disorder

72. A 34-year-old woman takes her 8-year-old daughter to a physician's office. She says that the child often experiences episodes of severe dyspnea and abdominal pain. The child's medical records shows many office visits and four abdominal surgical procedures that resulted in a "grid abdomen" due to crossed surgical scarring, although no abnormalities were ever found. When she is confronted with the doctor's suspicion that illness in the child is being faked by the mother, the mother angrily grabs the child and immediately leaves the office.

Diagnostic impression:

A) Factitious disorder by proxy
B) Malingering
C) Folie a deux
D) La belle indifference
E) Body dysmorphic disorder

73. A 48-year-old man claims that he injured his back at work. He asserts that his injury prevents him from working and interferes with his marital relationship. He has no further sign of back problems after he receives a $50,000 worker's compensation settlement, but still does not return to work.

Diagnostic impression:

A) Malingering
B) Factitious disorder
C) Pain disorder
D) Conversion disorder
E) Adjustment disorder

Medtext Medical World, Inc.

74.   A 20-year-old soldier cannot recall the events of a battle in which one half of his platoon was killed.

Diagnostic impression:

A) Dissociative fugue
B) Dissociative amnesia
C) Dissociative identity disorder
D) Dissociative personality disorder
E) Depersonalization disorder

75.   The medical differential diagnosis for dissociative disorders includes:

A) Substance abuse
B) Head injury
C) Delirium
D) Seizure disorder
E) All of the above

76.   A 32-year-old secretary who formerly lived in New York, has been to Oregon, and has been working as a cashier for more than 3 years. She has no memory of coming to Oregon or of living in New York.

Diagnostic impression:

A) Amnestic dissociation
B) Psychogenic fugue
C) Depersonality disorder
D) Dissociative identity disorder
E) Multiple personality disorder

77.	A 36-year-old woman is married, has two children, and usually dresses conservatively. She receives a letter containing a recent photograph of her in a low-cut sweater and a short skirt. She does not remember the man who wrote the letter. She has no recollection of purchasing the outfit or posing for the photograph.

Diagnostic impression:

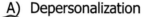

A)	Depersonalization
B)	Dissociative identity disorder
C)	Dissociative fugue
D)	Dissociative amnesia
E)	Borderline personality disorder

78.	A 40-year-old man says that he feels as if he is "outside himself" watching his life as though it were a movie. He knows that his perception is only a feeling and that he is really living his life.

Diagnostic impression:

A)	Depersonalization disorder
B)	Derealization disorder
C)	Prodrome to dissociative fugue
D)	Borderline personality disorder
E)	Dissociative personality disorder

79.	A 24-year-old woman experiences pelvic pain when she and her boyfriend attempt to have sexual intercourse. No abnormalities are found during pelvic examination.

Diagnostic impression:

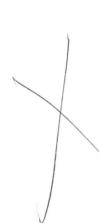

A)	Vaginismus
B)	Dyspareunia
C)	Orgasmic disorder
D)	Female arousal disorder
E)	Sexual aversion disorder

Medtext Medical World, Inc.

80. A 27-year-old couple married for 4 years have never had sexual intercourse because the wife has vaginal muscle spasms which prevent the husband from achieving vaginal penetration even though he has a full erection.

Although examination of the woman's external genitalia shows no abnormalities, a speculum cannot be readily inserted into the vagina (because of muscle contraction and pain).

Diagnostic impression:

A) Dyspareunia
B) Vaginismus
C) Orgasmic disorder
D) Hypoactive sexual desire
E) Sexual aversion disorder

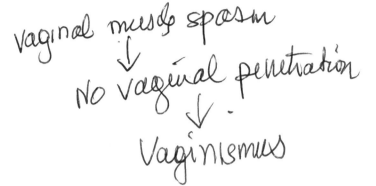

81. A 32-year-old man says that he usually has an orgasm and ejaculates before he achieves vaginal penetration.

Diagnostic impression:

A) Premature ejaculation
B) Orgasmic disorder
C) Male erectile disorder
D) Sexual aversion disorder
E) Gender dysphoria

82. Although she reports that she is sexually aroused, a 39-year-old woman has never reached orgasm by any means – during sexual activity with her husband, with a stimulation device, or during masturbation.

Diagnostic impression:

A) Sexual aversion disorder
B) Dyspareunia
C) Vaginismus
D) Orgasmic disorder
E) Hypoactive sexual desire

83.	A 39-year-old man (who has never before had problems with erections) begins to have difficulty achieving an erection during sexual activity with his wife. The first time he had trouble maintaining an erection was at a beach party when he had "too much to drink." He now has problems even when he does not drink.

Diagnostic impression:

A)	Sexual aversion disorder
B)	Dyspareunia
C)	Orgasmic disorder
D)	Hypoactive sexual desire
E)	Impotence

84.	A 32-year-old woman reports that although she is interested in engaging in sexual interaction with her husband (whom she describes as a patient, sensitive lover), she does not become physically aroused during their sexual activity.

Diagnostic impression:

A)	Sexual aversion disorder
B)	Female sexual arousal disorder
C)	Hypoactive sexual desire
D)	Dyspareunia
E)	Orgasmic disorder

85.	A 23-year-old woman (who does not have lesbian interests) enjoys dating men, but dislikes all sexual activity with them, including kissing.

Diagnostic impression:

A)	Hypoactive sexual desire
B)	Sexual aversion disorder
C)	Hypersexual avoidance syndrome
D)	Borderline personality
E)	Schizoid personality disorder

Medtext Medical World, Inc.

86. A 44-year-old man who has been married for 20 years says that although he still loves his wife, he no longer feels much desire to have sex with her or with anyone else.

    Diagnostic impression:

    A) Hypoactive sexual desire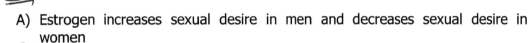
    B) Sexual aversion
    C) Hyporgasmic disorder
    D) Male erectile disorder
    E) Paraphilia

87. **True** of gonadal hormones in human sexuality:

    A) Estrogen increases sexual desire in men and decreases sexual desire in women
    B) Progesterone decreases sexual desire in both men and women
    C) Testosterone levels are increased by stress in men
    D) Testosterone has no impact on sexual desire
    E) Progesterone increases testosterone secretion

88. A 33-year-old woman says that she has always felt as if she was "a man in the body of a woman." She hates her breasts and feels as if her genitals do not belong to her. She is sexually attracted to heterosexual women, is most comfortable wearing men's clothing, and wants to take male hormones and undergo a mastectomy and surgical sex reversal so that she can live as a man.

    True of transsexuality:

    A) Differential diagnosis includes obsessive-compulsive disorder and body dysmorphism.
    B) Gender identity disorder is equally common among men and women.
    C) Prenatal etiology for gender identity disorder has been suggested.
    D) Cognitive therapy and cognitive-behavioral therapy is more efficacious than supportive psychotherapy.
    E) Sexual reorientation surgery is the preferred treatment.

Medtext Medical World, Inc.

89.   **TRUE** of homosexuality:

   A) Is more common in lower socioeconomic classes
   B) Is a normal variant of sexual expression
   C) Distress about one's sexual preference is no longer considered a dysfunction
   D) Most gay and lesbian people have not experienced heterosexual sex, and few have had children
   E) Homosexuality is more common but less public in women

90.   A 19-year-old gymnast says that she needs to lose 15 pounds to pursue a career in sports. She is 5 feet, 7 inches tall and weighs 95 pounds. Her mood is good. Findings on physical examination are normal except for excessive growth of downy body hair. She reports that she has not menstruated in more than 1 year.

   Diagnostic impression:

   A) Anorexia nervosa
   B) Body dysmorphic disorder
   C) Bulimia nervosa
   D) Obsessive compulsive personality disorder
   E) Narcissistic personality disorder

91.   A 22-year-old medical student has a parotid gland abscess. She is of normal weight for her height, but seems distressed when you question her about her eating habits.

   Diagnostic impression:

   A) Body dysmorphic disorder
   B) Anorexia nervosa
   C) Bulimia
   D) Avoidant personality disorder
   E) Social phobia

Medtext Medical World, Inc.

92. A 30-year-old professional ice skater is caught taking an inexpensive radio from a store without paying for it. He has been caught shoplifting twice before.

Diagnostic impression:

    A) Antisocial personality disorder
    B) Malingering
    C) Mania
    D) Kleptomania ✓
    E) Stealing for gain

93. A 34-year-old man is arrested for leaving his car and physically attacking another motorist stopped at a traffic light. A witness reports that the victim had cut the man off at the previous light.

Diagnostic impression:

    A) Alcohol or drug intoxication
    B) Dementia or psychosis
    C) Antisocial personality disorder
    D) Amok
    E) Intermittent explosive disorder

94. A 29-year-old woman wears a wig because she has pulled out all of the hair on the back of her head.

Diagnostic impression:

    A) Alopecia
    B) Obsessive-compulsive disorder
    C) Trichophagia
    D) Trichotillomania ✓
    E) Bipolar disorder, manic episode

Medtext Medical World, Inc.

95.   A 60-year-old woman is afraid to tell her husband that her credit cards are at their maximum because she lost more than $10,000 gambling in a casino. She ran up debt in this way twice before.

Diagnostic impression:

A) Pathological gambling
B) Gambling dependence
C) Gambling abuse
D) Manic episode
E) Impulse control disorder, not otherwise specified

96.   Six months after a mastectomy, a 48-year-old woman feels sad for a few minutes each evening and often wakes before her alarm goes off; however, she continues to do well in her job and enjoys social interactions with coworkers and family.

Diagnostic impression:

A) Body dysmorphic disorder
B) Acute stress disorder
C) Bereavement
D) Adjustment disorder
E) None of the above

97.   Four months after his parent's divorce, a 10-year-old boy seems sad at home most of the time, loses interest in playing with his friends, and begins to do poorly in school.

Diagnostic impression:

A) Adjustment disorder 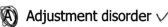 ✓
B) Normal grief reaction
C) Acute stress disorder
D) Major depression
E) Dysthymia

Medtext Medical World, Inc.

98. A 45-year-old hospital aide says that she was laid off because she worked too hard and made her supervisor look lazy. She says that when the same thing happened in a previous job, she filed a lawsuit against the hospital.

Diagnostic impression:

A) Paranoid personality disorder
B) Narcissistic personality disorder
C) Borderline personality disorder
D) Manic grandiosity
E) Obsessive compulsive personality disorder

99. The parents of a 28-year-old man say that they are concerned about him because he has no friends and spends most of his time hiking in the woods. You examine him and find that he is content with his solitary life and has no evidence of a formal thought disorder.

Diagnostic impression:

A) Schizotypal personality disorder
B) Schizoid personality disorder
C) Antisocial personality disorder
D) Dysthymia
E) Passive personality disorder

100. A 32-year-old woman says that her husband is angry because she calls him at the office many times each day to ask him to make trivial everyday decisions for her.

Diagnostic impression:

A) Dependent personality disorder
B) Folie a deux
C) Agoraphobia
D) Obsessive compulsive personality disorder
E) Obsessive compulsive disorder

101. A 28-year-old man comes to your office dressed in a black velvet beret and a cape lined with red satin. He reports that his mild sore throat felt like a "red hot poker" when he swallowed and says that he feels so warm that he "must have a fever of at least 106."

Diagnostic impression:

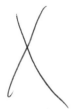

   A) Narcissistic personality disorder
   B) Schizotypal personality disorder
   C) Histrionic personality disorder
   D) Borderline personality disorder
   E) Hypochondriasis

102. A 33-year-old man reports that each night he created a detailed schedule of his activities for the next day. He tells you that his wife of 6 months recently moved out because she could not conform to his rigid rules.

Diagnostic impression:

   A) Obsessive compulsive disorder
   B) Narcissistic personality disorder
   C) Obsessive compulsive personality disorder
   D) Manic depressive disorder
   E) Relational disturbance, not otherwise specified

103. A 35-year-old man brags that he has been sexually assaulting women ever since high school, but has never been caught. He has often been unemployed and has been arrested for shoplifting several times.

Diagnostic impression:

   A) Antisocial personality disorder
   B) Narcissistic personality disorder
   C) Sexual deviant disorder
   D) Paraphilia, not otherwise specified
   E) Conduct disorder

Medtext Medical World, Inc.

104.   An oddly dressed 32-year-old woman says that she likes to walk in the woods because the birds communicate with her. She says that she never goes out on Thursdays, however, because they are "dangerous days." She has few friends.

Diagnostic impression:

    A) Schizoid personality disorder
    B) Schizotypal personality disorder ✓
    C) Schizophrenia, undifferentiated type
    D) Avoidant personality disorder
    E) Antisocial personality disorder

105.   A 38-year-old man asks you to refer him to a physician who attended a top medical school. He says that he knows you will not be offended because you understand that he is "better" than your other patients.

Diagnostic impression:

    A) Borderline personality disorder
    B) Narcissistic personality disorder
    C) Obsessive compulsive personality disorder
    D) Manic phase of bipolar disorder
    E) Factitious disorder

106.   A 35-year-old woman who works as a laboratory assistant lives with her elderly mother and rarely socializes. She reports that when coworkers ask her to join them for lunch, she refuses because she is afraid that they will not like her.

Diagnostic impression:

    A) Borderline personality disorder
    B) Narcissistic personality disorder
    C) Avoidant personality disorder
    D) Dependent personality disorder
    E) Passive aggressive personality disorder

107. A 21-year-old female college student tells you that because she was afraid to be alone again, she tried to commit suicide after a man with whom she had had two dates did not call her again. After your interview, she tells you that all of the other doctors she has seen were terrible and that you are the only doctor who has ever understood her problems.

Diagnostic impression:

A) Narcissistic personality disorder
B) Borderline personality disorder
C) Passive aggressive personality disorder
D) Hypomania
E) Dependent personality disorder

108. Two weeks after a 50-year-old overweight, hypertensive woman agreed to start an exercise program, she gained 4 pounds. She reports that she has not exercised yet because "the gym was so crowded that I couldn't get in."

Diagnostic impression:

A) Borderline personality disorder
B) Histrionic personality disorder
C) Narcissistic personality disorder
D) Avoidant personality disorder
E) Passive-aggressive personality disorder

109. **True** of steroid hormones:

A) Use of corticosteroids is associated with depression, confusion, psychotic symptoms and fatigue
B) Abrupt withdrawal of corticosteroids is associated with hypomania and euphoria
C) Thyroid supplements are associated with depression and fatigue
D) Progestins are associated anxiety and psychotic symptoms
E) Androgens are associated with aggressiveness and agitation

110. **True** of antihypertensives:

A) Severe depression and confusion is associated with reserpine
B) Fatigue and depression and uncommonly psychosis are associated with clonidine and methyldopa *mild depression fatigue + sexual dysfunction*
C) Verapamil are associated with anxiety and visual distortions —*depression*
D) Beta blockers are associated with anxiety and euphoria —*depression + fatigue*
E) Nifedipine has been associated with psychosis—*depression*

111. **True** of antibiotics:

A) Antituberculin drugs have been associated with confusion, headache and sleepiness —*memory loss + psychosis*
B) Nitrofurantoin has been associated with depression
C) Chloramphenicol is associated with depression, confusion, and irritability *and Flagyl*
D) Tetracycline is associated with anxiety —*depression*
E) Metronidazole is associated with anorexia and bulimia —*depression-*

112. **True** of analgesics:

A) Pentazocine has been associated with psychosis
B) Propoxyphene has been associated with paresthesias — *psychosis*
C) Salicylates have been associated with confusion, dizziness, psychotic symptoms, depression (less common) *euphoria —depression + confusion*
D) Indomethacin has been associated with euphoria, depression and confusion (in very high doses) *confusion —dizziness*
E) Phenylbutazone is associated with depression *anxiety*

113. **True** of patients undergoing renal dialysis:

A) Patients on renal dialysis are at increased risk for psychological problems, in part because they must depend on other people and on machines
B) Anxiety, psychosis and aggression are the most common psychological problems in renal dialysis patients
C) Medical risks are increased with in-home dialysis
D) Psychological risks are increased with in-home dialysis
E) In-home dialysis greatly disrupts a stable home life

114. Established reasons for psychological risk in patients with AIDS:

   A) The illness is potentially fatal
   B) Guilt for past high-risk behaviors
   C) Guilt for exposure of others to the virus
   D) Forced to 'come out" to others if homosexual
   E) All of the above

115. A 26-year-old man who has taken an antidepressant for 2 months comes to the emergency room with elevated blood pressure, sweating, headache, and vomiting. At a party he ate pizza that contained aged Parmesan cheese and drank punch that contained red wine.

   The antidepressant is:

   A) Phenelzine
   B) Citalopram
   C) Bupropion
   D) Venlafaxine
   E) Mirtazapine

116. Foods rich in tyramine include:

   A) Aged cheese
   B) Chicken or beef liver
   C) Smoked or pickled meat or fish
   D) Beer or red wine
   E) All of the above

117. Adverse effects associated with lithium include:

   A) Aplastic anemia
   B) Psychomotor slowing
   C) Liver toxicity
   D) Ebstein's anomaly
   E) Neural tube defects

118. Adverse effects associated with valproic acid:

    A) Congenital neural tube defects ✓
    B) Psychomotor slowing
    C) Sedation
    D) Renal dysfunction
    E) Thyroid dysfunction

119. Adverse effects associated with carbamazepine:

    A) Aplastic anemia
    B) Neural tube defects
    C) Alopecia
    D) Hypothyroidism.
    E) Renal dysfunction.

120. Adverse effects associated with topiramate:

    A) Psychomotor slowing *& fatigue*
    B) Dizziness
    C) Ataxia
    D) Blood dyscrasia
    E) Autoinduction

121. Adverse side effects associated with oxcarbazepine:

    A) Dizziness, ataxia, visual disturbances
    B) Blood dyscrasia
    C) Autoinduction
    D) Cardiac conduction disturbance
    E) Mild renal impairments

Medtext Medical World, Inc.

122. A 32-year-old woman on an antidepressant complains of Parkinsonian symptoms, galactorrhea, and sexual dysfunction. Her pharmacist warned her that this antidepressant was the most dangerous in overdose.

The antidepressant is:

A) Amoxapine
B) Bupropion
C) Mirtazapine
D) Tranylcypromine
E) Venlafaxine

123. Effects associated with bupropion:

A) Hypersomnolence → *Insomnia*
B) Seizures
C) Increased appetite — *↓ appetite*
D) Serotonin syndrome *NO*
E) Priapism — *NO Trazodone*

Refractory Depress
Indication: Fastest working SSRI within 10 days

124. Effects associated with venlafaxine:

A) Increased diastolic blood pressure
B) Lower remission rates — *highest remission rate + low sexual S/E*
C) Decreased appetite — *Bupropion*
D) Parkinsonian effects — *Amoxapine*
E) Orthostatic hypotension → *MAOI*

125. Indications for selective serotonin reuptake inhibitors (SSRIs) include all **EXCEPT**:

A) Obsessive compulsive disorder
B) Premature ejaculation
C) Premenstrual dysphoric disorder
D) Hypochondriasis
E) Impotence

Medtext Medical World, Inc.

126. **TRUE** of selective serotonin reuptake inhibitors:

    [handwritten: 70/08]

    A) Escitalopram has the highest incidence of gastrointestinal side effects ✓
    B) Paroxetine is associated with least amount of sexual dysfunction – .
    C) Citalopram is currently only indicated for obsessive compulsive disorder
    D) Fluvoxamine is associated with agitation and insomnia *[handwritten: —only OCD]*
    E) Fluoxetine is associated with sexual dysfunction *[circled]*

127. **TRUE** of the heterocyclic antidepressants:

    A) Clomipramine is the most noradrenergic and least sedating
    B) Nortriptyline is the most likely to cause orthostatic changes *[handwritten: → least likely to cause orthostatic change]*
    C) Maprotiline has low cardiotoxicity *[handwritten: → s/e seizures]* *[circled]*
    D) Imipramine is less likely to cause orthostatic changes *[handwritten: — more like to cause orthostatic change]*
    E) Amitriptyline is least anticholinergic *[handwritten: — more antich]*

    [handwritten: Desipramine least sedating - least anticholinergic]

128. Additional clinical indications for antipsychotic medications include:

    A) Perphenazine for body dysmorphic disorder
    B) Fluphenazine for non-psychotic anxiety
    C) Haloperidol for hiccups and emesis
    D) Trifluoperazine is available in long-acting (decanoate) form
    E) Olanzapine for negative symptoms *[circled]*

    [handwritten: Pimozine → Tourette + Body Dys. Dis]

129. Mature defense mechanisms include:

    A) Denial
    B) Projection
    C) Sublimation *[circled]*
    D) Splitting
    E) Lying

130. Although he was close to her, a man whose mother recently died describes the circumstances of her death dispassionately.

The defense mechanism described is:

A) Isolation of affect
B) Rationalization
C) Projection
D) Dissociation
E) Displacement

131. A job candidate who is not hired says, "I'm glad. That was a dead-end job anyway."

Defense mechanism described:

A) Isolation of affect
B) Rationalization
C) Help-rejecting complaining
D) Affiliation
E) Humor

132. A woman who has unacknowledged and unacceptable feelings for other men believes (without evidence) that her husband is cheating on her.

Defense mechanism described:

A) Defensive jealousy
B) Intellectualization
C) Projection
D) Anticipation
E) Acting out

133. In normal conversation with colleagues, a physician explains the technical details of the treatment options for his own terminal illness.

     Defense mechanism described:

     A) Sublimation
     B) Identification (with the aggressor)
     C) Tolerance
     D) Undoing
     E) Intellectualization

134. A man who was physically abused in childhood by his father abuses his own children.

     Defense mechanism described:

     A) Reaction formation
     B) Sublimation
     C) Identification
     D) Dissociation
     E) Idealization

135. A man who is uncomfortable with his baldness makes jokes about hair restoration techniques.

     Defense mechanism described:

     A) Humor
     B) Altruism
     C) Splitting
     D) Reaction negotiation
     E) Undoing

136. A surgical resident with unacknowledged anger toward her husband is abrasive to the male medical students on her service.

     Defense mechanism described:

     A) Suppression
     B) Displacement
     C) Regression
     D) Devaluation
     E) Self-assertion

137. An active 54-year-old woman insists that a laboratory report that shows that she has had a myocardial infarction is in error.

     Defense mechanism described:

     A) Denial
     B) Autistic fantasy
     C) Self-observation
     D) Self-accusation
     E) Self-initiation

138. A depressed 15-year-old boy with no history of conduct disorder steals a car after his parents separate.

     Defense mechanism described:

     A) Self-observation
     B) Omnipotence
     C) Passive aggression
     D) Misidentification of the aggression
     E) Acting out

Medtext Medical World, Inc.

139. A man with a poor self-image gives one-fifth of his annual salary to charity.

    Defense mechanism described:

    A) Self-assertion
    B) Help-rejecting complaining
    C) Projective identification
    D) Suppression
    E) Altruism

140. A man who is angry with his physician compliments her clothing.

    Defense mechanism described:

    A) Autistic fantasy
    B) Omnipotence
    C) Reaction formation
    D) Anticipation
    E) Devaluation

141. A woman who is hospitalized for minor surgery insists that her husband not leave her room.

    Defense mechanism described:

    A) Possessiveness
    B) Idealization
    C) Affiliation
    D) Passive aggression
    E) Regression

Medtext Medical World, Inc.

142. A physician becomes angry with a noncompliant patient who reminds her of her obstinate son.

Psychological phenomenon described:

  A) Transference
  B) Counter-transference
  C) Regression
  D) Repression
  E) Projection

143. A 30-year-old man with a mother who often disappointed him becomes angry when his physician attempts to terminate his consultation with her.

Psychological phenomenon described:

  A) Transference
  B) Projection
  C) Displacement
  D) Repression
  E) Regression

144. A hospitalized patient says that all of the weekday doctors are cold and insensitive, but that the weekend doctors are warm and friendly.

Defense mechanism described:

  A) Displacement
  B) Transference
  C) Counter-transference
  D) Splitting
  E) Undoing

Medtext Medical World, Inc.

145. A resident with strong destructive impulses chooses to do a residency in surgery.

   The defense mechanism described:

   A) Sublimation
   B) Suppression
   C) Undoing
   D) Reaction formation
   E) Transference

146. A woman who is diagnosed with terminal lung cancer as a result of smoking buys books on nutrition, stops smoking, and starts to exercise.

   Defense mechanism described:

   A) Suppression
   B) Sublimation
   C) Undoing
   D) Splitting
   E) Counter-transference

147. A 45-year-old man does not remember than he was sexually abused as a child.

   The defense mechanism described is:

   A) Sublimation
   B) Ego
   C) Repression
   D) Counter-transference
   E) Reaction formation

148.   Which of the following is present at birth and controlled by primary process thinking; contains instinctual sexual and aggressive drives?

    A) Id ✓

    B) Ego

    C) Superego

    D) Preconscious

    E) Unconscious

149.   Which of the following is developed by approximately 6 years of age?

    A) Id

    B) Ego

    C) Superego

    D) Preconscious

    E) Conscious

150.   A 45-year-old successful male attorney has been smoking on the average 10 cigarettes daily for 12 years. He has been recently diagnosed with a solitary coin lesion on CXR. He has had three previous failed attempts in smoking cessation. He has concerns that nicotine replacement therapy causes the same medical complications that are associated with smoking.

Select the **CORRECT** statement:

    A) He has a high degree of nicotine dependence

    B) Nicotine replacement therapy adversely affects cognition

    C) Nicotine replacement therapy does not cause acute vascular injury

    D) Bupropion combined with nicotine patch are unsafe

    E) Relaxing effects of smoking are lost with nicotine replacement therapy

Medtext Medical World, Inc.

151. A 21-year-old male with social phobia (social anxiety disorder) was recently divorced because his wife felt humiliated by his extreme shyness when she introduced him to her former high school classmates. He is currently seeking individual psychotherapy in order to gain control over his anxiety.

Which symptoms' cluster is common in social phobia?

A) Shyness persists despite attempts of self-medication with alcohol
B) Discrete episodes of anxiety are generalized to all social situations
C) Fears of being labeled as a "Psycho" is uncommon
D) It can precede substance abuse 85% of the time
E) Avoidant personality traits are uncommon

152. A 30-year-old woman taking disulfiram became pregnant. She is seeking advice about the effect of disulfiram on her pregnancy.

Which of the following statements is **MOST** correct?

A) The combination with alcohol has teratogenic effects
B) The combination with alcohol causes hypertension
C) The combination with alcohol increases placental perfusion
D) Disulfiram has antipsychotic effects
E) All of the above is correct

153. A 74-year-old man was recently diagnosed with Alzheimer's disease. He is willing to be treated with "anti-dementia medications." He has difficulty swallowing tablets and capsules.

Which of the following "anti-dementia medications" is available in an oral solution form?

A) Rivastigmine
B) Tacrine
C) Risperidone
D) Donepezil
E) None of the above

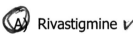
Liquid forme: Rivastigmine

154. A 50-year-old male housekeeper was stuck in the hotel elevator for two hours. The elevator telephone was out of service. He was extricated. He was noticed to be anxious, and was complaining of chest tightness and had profuse sweating. He was medically cleared and sent home. Later that night, he was unable to sleep. He experienced chest tightness, profuse sweating and began hearing the elevator alarm over and over again.

Which of the following symptoms meet the diagnostic criteria for Acute Stress Disorder?

A) He experienced intense fear in the elevator
B) Dissociative amnesia is uncommon
C) His disturbances must occur within 2 days of the incident
D) His disturbances cause a minor degree of distress
E) All of the above are correct criteria

155. A 35-year-old male patient with chronic paranoid schizophrenia has been treated in the past with thiothixene, haloperidol, olanzapine and risperidone. His care has been transferred to a mental health center with a restricted pharmacy formulary. He has been told that he can only receive antipsychotic medications that have been FDA- approved for the long-term treatment of schizophrenia.

Which of the following is **NOT** FDA- approved for the long-term treatment of schizophrenia?

A) Olanzapine
B) Ziprasidone
C) Risperidone
D) Clozapine
E) Aripiprazole

156. A 45-year-old single, female has been successfully treated for recurrent major depression with a 60 mg daily fluoxetine dose. She has been maintaining an ideal body weight through dieting and regular exercise. Over the last three months she has been gaining weight. She has been recently engaged and anticipating getting married within 6 months. She is concerned that her expensive wedding dress will not fit her.

Which of the following strategies can be **FIRST** considered to minimize antidepressant weight gain?

A) Fluoxetine dose reduction
B) Adjunctive treatment with bupropion
C) Fluoxetine switching
D) Adjunctive treatment with topiramate
E) Adjunctive treatment with a 5-HT 2C agonist

157. A 30-year-old male who uses cocaine daily, has recently been diagnosed with hypertension. He has family history of cerebrovascular accidents (CVA's) including myocardial infarctions and strokes.

Which of the following have been associated with cocaine use?

A) CVA's usually occur in patients in their mid 20's
B) Infarctions are more common than hemorrhages
C) Cocaine related CVA's are due to vasospasm
D) Pre-existing cerebral lesions were present in all cases
E) Cerebral hemisphere strokes are less common than brainstem infarctions

158. A 30-year-old male with the diagnosis of AIDS is being treated for pulmonary tuberculosis. He presented with recurrent generalized seizures that progressed into intractable seizures. He has also been drinking 36 cans of beer daily and has a history of alcohol withdrawal delirium.

Which of the following medications need to be considered immediately?

A) Fosphenytoin
B) Thiamine
C) Lorazepam
D) Pyridoxine
E) All of the above

159.   In the third year of a psychiatry residency training program, the child psychiatry rotation include a didactic course on Margaret Mahler early childhood relationships theory.

Which of the following statements apply to that theory?

A) Separation individuation phase occurs at 36 months.
B) Separation anxiety occurs between 10 and 16 months
C) Stranger anxiety occurs between 16 and 24 months
D) Rapprochement occurs between 24 and 36 months
E) All of the above

160.   A 45-year-old woman was involved in a motor vehicle accident. She did not lose consciousness. Neurological evaluation and brain imaging studies confirmed an orbitofrontal brain lesion.

What are the possible manifestations of such an injury?

A) Lack of distractibility
B) Euphoria
C) Apathy
D) Intact judgment
E) Increase remorse

161.   A hot air balloon rider had an emergency accelerated landing which led to a crash and to an open head injury. He experienced loss of consciousness. Following a protracted period of treatment and neurological rehabilitation, he developed a neuropsychiatric condition manifested by hypermetamorphosis

Which of the following conditions may also develop?

A) Hypersexuality
B) Hypophagia
C) Aggression
D) Anxiety
E) Phobias

162. Due to the influence of psychosocial sciences on the development of behavioral sciences, a psychiatry specialty oral board examiner is inquiring about such influences.

    Which of the following are accurate connections?

    A) Pavlov's concept of surrogate mother
    B) Harlow's study of Aphasia
    C) Kandel's concept of experimental neurosis
    D) Lorenz's concept of imprinting
    E) All of the above

163. A 61-year-old male car salesman with a recent cerebrovascular accident (CVA) developed left hemiparesis. He is concerned about his cognitive functioning.

    Which of the following are of concern?

    A) He may experience "visual non-verbal" task deficits
    B) Rehabilitation may improve his semantic memory
    C) He may experience a decline in episodic memory
    D) He may experience" auditory verbal" task deficits
    E) He may experience improvement in recent memory

164. A 24-year-old ecology student developed phobia to snakes .He won't be able to join his classmate on a much anticipated amazon forest expedition. He wants to understand the psychological defense mechanisms involved in the development of phobias.

    What is the **MAJOR** defense mechanism in phobia?

    A) Repression
    B) Displacement
    C) Controlling
    D) Abreaction
    E) Projection

Medtext Medical World, Inc.

165.   A child psychiatry fellow diagnosed a 10-year-old boy with one of the pervasive developmental disorder (PDD).

Which of the following features differentiate this PDD from Autistic disorder?

    A) The onset of the disorder is prior to age 3
    B) The male to female ratio is 1:1
    C) Approximately 75% of the children are mentally retarded
    D) The presence of normal language development
    E) The prevalence of the disorder is 2/10,000

166.   A 75-year-old woman became disoriented and confused following open heart surgery. A psychiatric consultation was conducted and documented the presence of delirium.

Which of the following is **TRUE** in regard to Delirium?

    A) Delirium is a prodrome for dementia
    B) Delirium incidence is unknown in surgical patients
    C) Delirium improves with ongoing sedation
    D) Delirium is aggravated with 1:1 observation
    E) Delirium agitation is reduced with midazolam

167.   A 70-year-old man with dementia of the Alzheimer's type (DAT) and history of cerebrovascular accident had a recent neurological evaluation. The neurologist raised some challenges to the DAT diagnosis.

Which of the following description is accurate?

    A) Vascular dementia account for 30% of dementia cases
    B) Lewy Bodies are present in 25% of dementia cases
    C) Neurofibrillary tangles of DAT contain Beta Amyloid
    D) Early age of onset has a better prognosis than late onset DAT
    E) Chromosomal mutations account for 15% of dementia cases

168. A child with mental retardation was diagnosed with Williams Syndrome.

What are the characteristic features of Williams Syndrome?

A) Comorbid ADHD — *Depression* — *Anxiety*
B) Comorbid OCD
C) Aortic dilatation → *Aortic stenosis*
D) Hypotension — *hypertension*
E) All of the above

169. A 7-year-old boy living in the Northeastern U.S.A was bitten by a tick. His parents are concerned about his risks of developing a tick-borne infectious disease.

Which of the following are present in that disease?

A) The organism can be identified by a specific laboratory test
B) Within hours flu-like symptoms will develop
C) Labile mood may be the initial presentation
D) Remission occur with appropriate treatment
E) The heart is among the target organs

170. A 73-year-old woman sustained a recent stoke with left hemiparesis. When her grandchildren visited her in the hospital she seemed aloof and unloving.

Which of the following is the **BEST** response?

A) Motor aprosodia is present
B) Sensory aprosodia is absent —
C) Blunted affect coincide with depression
D) It is a dominant hemisphere phenomenon *No*
E) All of the above are correct.

Non-dominant *Left*

171. A 35-year-old male with highly elevated liver enzymes refuse to receive treatment for alcohol dependence. He reports that alcohol is the most relaxing drug that he has ever had. He also fears that without alcohol use he will be a "nervous wreck".

The CNS effects of alcohol seem to be mediated by:

   A) Interaction with nor- adrenaline
   B) Activation of glutamate receptors.
   C) Release of dopamine
   D) Inhibition of opioid peptides
   E) All of the above

172. A psychiatry resident presents to his clinical supervisor the various psychotherapeutic modalities.

Which of the following associations are **CORRECT**?

   A) Anna Freud: Self-Psychology 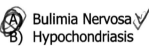 *Ego psychology*
   B) Isaac Mark: Interpersonal Psychotherapy
   C) Joseph Wolpe: Behavior Therapy
   D) Donald Winnicott: Psychodynamic Psychotherapy
   E) Heinz Kohut: Ego Psychology

173. A 45-year-old man is worried that his teen age daughter may follow his foot steps of chain smoking. He is considering hypnosis as a therapeutic intervention for smoking cessation.

Which types of clinical disorders respond **BEST** to hypnosis?

   A) Bulimia Nervosa
   B) Hypochondriasis
   C) Somatic delusion
   D) Heroin dependence
   E) Conversion disorder

Medtext Medical World, Inc.

174. A 55-year-old male with liver cirrhosis due to life long alcohol dependence is being considered for a liver transplant.

    What are the guidelines for selecting organ transplant recipients?

    A) Pediatric consideration can be delayed
    B) Psychiatric conditions are included
    C) Utilitarian-oriented position
    D) Ventilator-dependent patients are candidates
    E) Medical urgency may override the waiting list

175. A 75-year-old terminally ill woman with adenocarcinoma of the lungs has come to term in accepting her death.

    What are the **MOST** common fears associated with death?

    A) Death will cause suffocation
    B) Death will bring intense guilt
    C) Death will cause intense pain
    D) Death will result in abandonment
    E) All of the above

176. A 78-year-old male patient with the diagnosis of dementia not other wise specified (NOS) recently undergone a series of lumbar punctures (LP) to rule out possible central nervous system (CNS) infection due to recurrent urinary tract infections (UTI's.) His primary care physician was surprised to notice an improvement in his cognitive functioning following these LP's.

    Which of the following are typical of this condition?

    A) Visual hallucinations
    B) Auditory hallucinations
    C) Overflow incontinence
    D) Magnetic gait
    E) Fluctuation in cognition

    ~ Magnetic Gait
    ~ Incontinence
    — Dementia
    — Cognitive alleviate
    by Lumbar Punction

Medtext Medical World, Inc.

177. Due to some differences in the diagnostic criteria of dementia of the Alzheimer's type (DAT) between neurologists and psychiatrists, a dually certified neurology/psychiatry diplomate outlined to the medical students a criterion that does not provide an evidence for DAT.

Which of the following criteria did he outline?

    A) Memory impairment
    B) Apraxia
    C) Apathy
    D) Anhedonia
    E) Agnosia

178. A 26-year-old prison inmate with the diagnosis of antisocial personality disorder, methamphetamine dependence and impulse control disorder not otherwise specified (NOS) is illusive, unpredictable and verbally aggressive.

Which of the following is a potentially useful treatment?

    A) Dextroamphetamine
    B) Aversive techniques
    C) Mirtazapine therapy
    D) Anticonvulsive agents
    E) Dynamic psychotherapy

179. A 29-year-old female patient with borderline personality disorder felt dysphoric, abandoned and hopeless. She is being treated with escitalopram. She was also taking an old prescription of amitriptyline for sleep. Her neighbor offered her St John's Wort tea to help her relax at nighttime. She continued to drink that tea every night.

On a hot summer day she was found by her boyfriend laying on the floor, confused and complaining of "burning hot."

What are some of the characteristics of the syndrome that she may have developed?

    A) Hypotension
    B) Myoclonus
    C) Bradycardia
    D) Hypothermia
    E) All of the above

Serotonin syndrome char by: Hypertension – Tachycardia Hyperthermia

Medtext Medical World, Inc.

180. A 49-year-old female patient with bipolar disorder Type I and family history of nephrogenic diabetes insipidus (DI) responded well to lithium therapy. Her urinary output is 2.5L/Day.She refuses to consider alternative mood stabilizers.

Which statement is **MOST** accurate?

A) Polyuria occurs in most patients on long-term lithium therapy
B) Thiazide diuretics increase urine volume causing nephrogenic DI
C) She has already developed nephrogenic DI
D) Nephrogenic DI develops in 20% of lithium therapy
E) Single bedtime lowest effective lithium dose is recommended

181. A 24-year-old female has been repeatedly hospitalized for a recurrence of a physical symptom. She is preoccupied with her general state of health. She has exaggerated fears of having undiagnosed diseases.

What is the **MOST** probable diagnosis?

A) Histrionic personality
B) Somatization disorder
C) Factitious disorder
D) Somatic delusion
E) Hypochondriasis

182. An 18-year-old adolescent boy attempted suicide by overdosing on an unknown amount of a white powder. He appeared flighty and euphoric. His girlfriend believes that it was crack.

What are the acute effects of crack?

A) Bradycardia
B) Hyperphagia
C) Decreased alertness
D) Increased sexual excitement
E) Relaxation

     Medtext Medical World, Inc.

183. Mental retardation (MR) is a condition with diverse causes. Some cases of MR have no clear etiology. There are common causes of MR that account for 30% of identified cases.

Which of the following are common causes of MR?

A) Prader. Willis Syndrome
B) Copraxia
C) Fragile X Syndrome
D) Williams Syndrome
E) Stereotype

184. A 72-year-old woman with Parkinson's disease is referred for transcranial magnetic stimulation (TMS) treatment.

Which of the following brain location has been identified as the **BEST** site for treatment?

A) Substantia nigra
B) Subthalamic nucleus
C) Anterior putamen
D) Ventral lateral thalamic nucleus
E) None of the above

185. A Family Medicine resident is in the process of preparing for his specialty board examination. He asked his friend who is a Psychiatry resident about the most appropriate agent to treat anticholinergic drug toxicity.

What would the Psychiatry resident recommend?

A) Physostigmine
B) Atropine
C) Propranolol
D) Clonazepam
E) Benztropine

186. In an introductory biostatistics course, the instructor is explaining to the students the appropriate question that can be answered by conducting a case-control study.

    A student with a degree in public health would chose which answer?

    A) Designed for prospective studies
    B) Designed to investigate a particular disease
    C) Designed to provide a prevalence rate
    D) Designed for diseases with low incidence ✓
    E) Designed as a clinical case trial

187. A 35-year-old African American male, is receiving various medications for treatment of diabetes, hypertension, and tension headache.

    Which of the following medications has nearly no effects on inhibiting the 1A2, 3A4, 2C9, 2C19 and 2D6 of the P450 isoenzymes system?

    A) Clomipramine
    B) Fluoxetine
    C) Fluvoxamine
    D) Citalopram
    E) Paroxetine

188. A psychotherapist, who specializes in long-term dynamic psychotherapy, is changing his practice to short-term dynamic psychotherapy to meet his HMO new reimbursement regulations.

    Which of the following will characterize his newly referred patients?

    A) Lack of psychological mindedness
    B) No past meaningful relationships
    C) Establishment of a psychotherapeutic focus ✓
    D) Unknown duration of treatment
    E) Absence of flexible defenses

189. A 16-year-old boy had a sore throat which tested positive for group A beta-hemolytic streptococcus infection.

    What are the possible psychiatric sequelae of this infection?

    A) Depression NOS
    B) Psychotic disorder NOS
    C) Mania
    D) Obsessive-compulsive disorder
    E) Any of the above

190. A high school student enrolled in a military academy has ongoing conflicts with one of his instructors. He reported to the school commander that, although "he harbors no resentment, he is deeply convinced that this instructor despises him".

    What does the student's statement reflect?

    A) Reaction formation
    B) Displacement
    C) Rationalization
    D) Projection
    E) Repression

191. A jeweler from an Asian descent was invited to a Halloween party. He felt nauseated and noticed that he had a cutaneous rash. A paramedic attending the same party examined him and found him to be tachycardic and hypotensive.

    The jeweler most probably used:

    A) Inhalent
    B) Steroid
    C) Opioid
    D) Alcohol
    E) Methamphetamine

192. A popular singer received negative publicity following a concert in which he was unable to complete some of his songs. He later realized that this was due to his inability to swallow his saliva. A neurological evaluation confirmed the diagnosis of Amyotrophic lateral sclerosis (ALS) familial type.

Which gene mutation has been implicated in familial ALS?

A) Superoxide dismutase (SOD)
B) Cytoskeletal protein
C) LIM kinase -1 gene
D) Beta-globin gene
E) Beta-amyloid precursor protein (BAPP)

ALS → SOD

193. A 23-year-old woman with borderline personality disorder (BPD) has recurrence of suicidal acts by overdosing on non-lethal amounts of over the counter cold medications.

Which type of psychotherapy has been designed to decrease BPD suicidal acts?

A) Interpersonal therapy
B) Dialectical therapy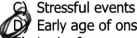
C) Cognitive behavioral therapy
D) Brief psychotherapy
E) Dynamic psychotherapy

194. A 19-year-old male who was adopted at birth was hospitalized for a first psychotic break. Some adoption medical records suggest that one of his biological parents was diagnosed with schizophrenia.

Which of the following has been associated with a poor prognosis in schizophrenia?

A) Paranoid delusions
B) Family history of mania
C) Stressful events
D) Early age of onset
E) Lack of expressed emotions

195. A 75-year-old woman with Parkinson's disease is likely to exhibit which of the following symptoms.

   A) A resting tremor ✓
   B) An action tremor
   C) An intention tremor
   D) A sad affect
   E) A senile tremor

196. A 32-year-old laboratory technician diagnosed with diabetes Type II, developed peripheral neuropathy. He asked his primary care provider to prescribe him an antidepressant for treatment of his neuropathy. He wants this antidepressant to have reliable therapeutic blood levels.

   Which antidepressant has clinically useful blood levels?

   A) Amitriptyline
   B) Sertraline
   C) Doxepin
   D) Nortriptyline
   E) Trazodone

197. The National Institute of Mental Health (NIMH) landmark Epidemiologic Catchment Area (ECA) has documented that the lifetime rates of antisocial personality disorder have been found to be:

   A) Highest among African Americans
   B) Lowest among Caucasian non-Hispanics
   C) Lowest among Asians
   D) Highest among Hispanics
   E) None of the above

Medtext Medical World, Inc.

198. A 25-year-old female student with multiple sclerosis (MS) is choosing a career in estate planning. She was referred by her teacher to a psychologist for a Wisconsin Card Sorting Test.

Which of the following items are best assessed by the Wisconsin Card Sorting Test?

A) Executive functioning
B) Abstract reasoning
C) Fluid memory
D) Crystallized memory
E) Emotional intelligence

199. Tom is a 44-year-old Caucasian assistant bank manager working in the Midwest when he became, "weak in the knees." Tom was diagnosed with multiple sclerosis; and, for a short time seemed to improve, but still had difficulty walking. Tom had to discontinue his daily "treadmill walks," because he could not keep his balance on his treadmill. Tom wants to know his prognosis.

You tell Tom that his outlook is:

A) Great
B) Reasonably good
C) Difficult to say
D) Unfavorable
E) Ghastly

200. Ellen is a 32-year-old Ph.D. candidate in computer engineering who has just been diagnosed with multiple sclerosis. She has completed all of her graduate work and is now having difficulty preparing for the first defense of her thesis.

Which of the following **MIGHT** be present?

A) Problems with concentration
B) Problems with attention
C) Problems with recent memory
D) Problems with information processing
E) All of the above

---

201. Which of the following is the metabolic precursor of dopamine used to treat Parkinson's Disorder?

   A) Lidocaine
   B) Levodopa
   C) Lithium
   D) Lamivudine
   E) None of the above

202. Karen is a 60-year-old District Attorney (D.A.) facing early retirement with early Parkinson's disorder. She inquires, "If I take levodopa, what is the probability of my developing side effects?"

   You answer:

   A) 20%
   B) 40%
   C) 60%
   D) 80%
   E) 90%

203. Susan is a 39-year-old high school basketball coach and physical fitness enthusiast who is into health foods and herbal remedies. When Susan is brought to the emergency department in a semi-obtunded encephalopathic state with no fever, and no localizing or lateralizing neurologic signs, what quick, simple, inexpensive, risk-free test might be a clue to the diagnosis of (herbal-induced) lead intoxication?

   A) Basophilic stippling of her red blood cells
   B) Magnetic Resonance Imaging of her brain (M.R.I.)
   C) Computerized Axial Tomography (C.T. scan)
   D) Electroencephalogram (E.E.G.)
   E) Electromyogram (E.M.G.)

204. Marsha is 18-years-old. Her father Jack is 41-years-old. Her grandfather Sam is 82-years-old. Her mother Sarah is 39-years-old. All drive motor vehicles.

Who would be expected to have the **HIGHEST** driver fatality rates?

    A) Marsha
    B) Jack
    C) Sam and Marsha   −18/82
    D) Jack and Sarah
    E) Sarah

205. Meningiomas are what percentage of the incidental tumors found at autopsy?

    A) 10%
    B) 20%
    C) 30%
    D) 40%
    E) 50%

206. John is 2-years-old. Bobby is 14-years-old. William is 44-years-old. Jill is 62-years-old, and Howard is 60-years-old.

Who is **MOST** likely to present with an intracranial meningioma?

    A) John
    B) Bobby
    C) William
    D) Jill
    E) Howard

D - Jill 62 yo

207. Jill, a 57-year-old professor of chemical engineering, presents with facial pain and anesthesia (Vth cranial nerve damage), visual impairment due to compression of her optic nerve and with extra-ocular muscle impairment due to palsy of her III, IV, and VI cranial nerves.

You would anticipate her brain tumor to be located in:

A) Sphenoidal wing
B) Parasagittal area
C) Olfactory grove
D) Suprasellar area
E) Infratentorial area

[handwritten: Partial seizures + leg weakness]
[handwritten: Loss of sense of smell Anosmia and reduce intellectual functioning ie Dementia]
[handwritten: bitemporal Hemianopsia]
[handwritten: Headache - Vertigo + Ataxia]

208. Meningiomas are histopathologically:

A) Benign
B) Malignant
C) Predominantly benign but may be atypically malignant
D) Malignant in adults and benign in children
E) Predominantly malignant but may be atypically benign

209. Mary and Jack are both police officers have been married for six years. They have two children Keisha, 3-years-old and Elijah, 18-months-old. While off-duty, Jack entered a convenience store to buy milk while a robbery was in progress. Jack identified himself as a police officer, drew his weapon, and when one perpetrator fired and missed, Jack fired and killed one perpetrator with one shot. Another perpetrator entered the store behind Jack; fired twice and hit Jack twice in his back. Jack died instantly.

The ways in which Mary **MAY** express may her anger might well include:

A) Screaming
B) Throwing objects
C) Striking objects
D) Striking others
E) All of the above

Medtext Medical World, Inc.

210. You are paged STAT to the Emergency Room as the consultation-liaison psychiatrist. Pandemonium reigns. Jack's body is on a gurney covered with a sheet. Mary, a second-degree black belt in Tae-Kwon-Do, has just kicked two nursing assistants in the groin. Mary is surrounded by five hospital staff ready to place her in leather restraints. A police marksman is outside ready to enter the emergency room. Keisha and Elijah are shrieking.

You should **NOT** say:

A) God never gives us more than we can handle
B) Only the good die young
C) Aren't you lucky that at least you were married for six years with children?
D) You must be strong for your children
E) All of the above

211. Mary's crisis continues. Keisha and Elijah are still shrieking.

You **MAY** say

A) I cannot imagine how difficult this is for you
B) I know this is very painful for you
C) It is harder, much harder than most people think
D) It is O.K. to be angry with God
E) All of the above

212. Sally a 27-year-old certified public accountant and John a 31-year-old tax attorney in pre-marital counseling for 3 weeks both use their cellular phones constantly and both worry if they might develop a brain tumor from their cellular phones.

You endorse:

A) Cellular phones have been associated with brain tumors
B) Cellular phones sometimes cause brain tumor
C) Cellular phones are dangerous only in certain geographic locations
D) Cellular phones are dangerous only during certain times of the day
E) Cellular phones are not associated with brain tumors

Medtext Medical World, Inc.

213. Diane, a 38-year-old industrial engineer, reports that she underwent hysterectomy and bilateral oophorectomy for ovarian carcinoma and is now receiving estrogen replacement therapy. She reports that prior to her surgery she was generally orgasmic and frequently multiorgasmic. Now she reports that she is rarely initiates sexual activity and rarely is orgasmic and is no longer multiorgasmic and is requesting treatment.

Which of the following are **MOST** likely to restore her libido and her orgasms?

A) Fluoxetine (Prozac)
B) Sertraline (Zoloft)
C) Paroxetine (Paxil)
D) Testosterone
E) Estrogen

214. Four months have passed. Diane is now pleased with her sexual activity. Diane once again initiates sex with her husband and is now generally orgasmic and occasionally multiorgasmic. Diane is concerned about her new growth of facial hair.

You recommend:

A) Depilatories
B) Electrolysis
C) Shaving
D) Flornithine hydrochloride (Veniqua)
E) All of the above

215. In marital therapy with John a 34-year-old architect, Jane a 32-year-old commercial artist, endorses, "I rarely achieve orgasm during sex doctor!"

You inform Jane (and John) that:

A) Most women are not consistently orgasmic with penile-vaginal intercourse
B) A program of directed masturbation has been shown to be effective for woman with female orgasmic disorder
C) Women exhibit great variability in the type and intensity of stimulation required to trigger an orgasm
D) Couple therapy that focuses on communication skills has been shown to be effective
E) All of the above

Medtext Medical World, Inc.

216. Susan, a 31-year-old National Park Ranger, newly married for the first time, inquires in therapy, "Will I be able to continue my anti-depressant if I become a nursing mother?"

     You inform Susan that:

     A) All anti-depressants are safe for nursing mothers
     B) All anti-depressants are unsafe for nursing mothers
     C) Uncertain if anti-depressants are unsafe for nursing mothers
     D) Check with your Pediatrician
     E) Check with your OB-GYN

217. Carla, a 30-year-old: military aviator is grounded because of 60 days of repeated, unprovoked, sudden vomiting. Carla's neurologist finds no localizing or lateralizing neurologic signs and no pathologic reflexes. Carla's neurologist orders no tests because Carla has no headache and no papilledema. Carla's gastroenterologist finds nothing abnormal on her esophagogastroduodenoscopy. Carla's OB-GYN finds a negative pregnancy test and a normal pelvic examination. Carla endorses, "Now they are sending me to a psychiatrist because they think it is all in my head!"

     You recommend:

     A) Psychodynamic psychotherapy
     B) Magnetic Resonance Imaging
     C) A vacation for a full three months
     D) Military retirement
     E) Permanent grounding with no further duty as an aviator

218. Laura, a 34-year-old associate professor of Mathematics has been dating William, a 37-year-old associate professor of English Literature. Laura endorses in pre-marital therapy, "I know that William has been addicted to heroin. Now that William has been through a rehabilitation program and had been clean and sober for 3 years, what is his prognosis doctor?"

     You endorse:

     A) Ten years after heroin rehabilitation, 15% die
     B) Twenty years after heroin rehabilitation, 30% die
     C) Thirty years after heroin rehabilitation, 50% die
     D) All of the above
     E) None of the above

219. Laura further inquires, "Doctor, what is the probability that William is still using heroin?"

You endorse:

A) 10%
B) 20%
C) 30%
D) 40%
E) 50%

220. Laura inquires, "William has been clean and sober for 5 years. Doctor what is the probability that he will remain clean and sober for 5 more years?"

You respond:

A) 10%
B) 20%
C) 30%
D) 40%
E) 50%

221. Recent research has identified a second center in the rat brain; that, in addition to the "dopamine-rich" reward center in the rat forebrain, can trigger new drug craving.

This rat brain second center is located in the:

A) Hippocampus
B) Amygdala
C) Medulla Oblongata
D) All of the above
E) None of the above

222. Jill, a 48-year-old architect, Jane a 44-year-old attorney, Bill an 82-year-old retired shoe salesman, Esther a 31-year-old restaurant manager, and Sally, a 23-year-old college junior all live in the same neighborhood.

Who is **MOST** at risk for the development of pathological gambling?

A) Jill
B) Jane
C) Bill   82 y. o
D) Esther
E) Sally

223. Which of the following makes gambling pathological?

A) Persistent gambling
B) Recurrent gambling
C) Maladaptive gambling
D) All of the above
E) None of the above

224. The negative consequences of pathological gambling include:

A) Divorce
B) Job loss
C) Financial problems
D) Strained relationships
E) All of the above

225. Tom, a 58-year-old used car salesman is en route to Las Vegas. Tom endorses, "Doc, I just have to try to recoup my losses. Perhaps then, my wife, Sally, a 56-year-old waitress will take me back and then my kids won't be so ashamed of me!"

Tom's luck and his life are expected to:

A) Steadily improve
B) Steadily deteriorate
C) Stay about the same
D) Unpredictable
E) Win big this time!

226. Charles, an 82-year-old Professor Emeritus of Physics at the local university. Charles' family is requesting an evaluation for dementia as Charles is becoming increasingly forgetful; e.g. losing his house keys, forgetting his home address, and becoming, at times, angry at various members of his family. Charles is an active alcoholic. Charles attends AA but he drinks after the AA meetings. Charles' family inquires if Charles can be evaluated for dementia while he is actively drinking.

You respond:

A) Yes
B) No
C) Uncertain
D) All of the above
E) None of the above

227. Tim a 70-year-old Bank C.E.O. developed sudden loss of the use of his dominant right arm which cleared in 12 hours.

What is Tim's expected risk-of-stroke 18 months following his transient ischemic attack (T.I.A)?

A) 5%
B) 10%
C) 15%
D) 20%
E) 25%

---

228. Mental Status Testing includes:

A) Orientation
B) Recent and remote memory
C) Language
D) Apraxia (Inability to perform complex motor acts)
E) All of the above

229. Alzheimer's Disorder is responsible for what percentage of dementia cases?

A) 10-25%
B) 20-35%
C) 30-45%
D) 40-55%
E) 50-80%

230. John, a 55-year-old biomedical engineer, Mary, an 85-year-old high school dropout), Peter, a 60-year-old full professor of French Literature), Sam, a 48-year-old physicist, and Jack, a 41-year-old dentist are all your patients. None have a family history of Alzheimer's Disorder. None have any history of head trauma.

Who is at **GREATEST** risk of immediate Alzheimer's Disorder?

A) John
B) Mary → *Family H/o*
C) Peter   *Head Trauma*
D) Sam   *Female Sex*
E) Jack   *Advanced age*
             Lack of Education

Medtext Medical World, Inc.

231.	Mary, an 85-year-old high school dropout, goes on to develop Alzheimer's Disorder.

Which of the following **MIGHT** she develop in the intermediate stage of her disorder?

A) Capgras' syndrome
B) Encephalotrigeminal syndrome
C) Horner's syndrome
D) All of the above
E) None of the above

232.	Sharon a 57-year-old magazine editor has been married to Bill, a 59-year-old civil engineer for 33 years. Bill has been doing well following open heart surgery and quadruple vessel bypass 3 years ago. Bill collapses and dies suddenly and unexpectedly.

Which of the following **MAY** be anticipated in Sharon?

A) Avoidance
B) Numbness
C) Hyper-arousal
D) All of the above
E) None of the above

233.	In family therapy Sharon's daughter inquires, "If Bill had died after a prolonged illness might that have been easier for Sharon?"

You respond:

A) Yes
B) No
C) Varies with the length of the relationship
D) Varies with the occupation of the widow (or widower)
E) None of the above

234. Jim, a 34-year-old school bus driver, has been married to Elizabeth, a 31-year-old auto mechanic for 7 years. Elizabeth commits suicide by carbon monoxide inhalation.

What is Jim's risk of Post Traumatic Stress Disorder?

   A) 06%
   B) 16%
   C) 26%
   D) 36%
   E) 46%

235. Jim's family inquires, "Doctor how long will it take for Jim to "get over" this P.T.S.D?"

You respond:

   A) It varies with the age of the bereaved
   B) It varies with the occupation of the bereaved
   C) It varies with the gender of the bereaved
   D) It could well be a chronic illness for years
   E) He should be well in 60-90 days

236. Peter, 35-years-old, Paul, 37-years-old, Tom, 24-years-old, Vanessa 40-years-old, and Richard, 50-years old, all work at the same advertising agency.

By age alone, who is **MOST** probable to present at a Mental Health Clinic with Obsessive-Compulsive-Disorder (O.C.D)?

   A) Peter
   B) Paul
   C) Tom
   D) Vanessa
   E) Richard

237. Rorschach ink blot tests on Nazi war criminals post-W.W.II (after World War II) revealed:

   A) Chronic psychoses
   B) Chronic schizophrenia
   C) Chronic bipolar disorder
   D) Chronic obsessive compulsive disorder
   E) None of the above

238. Heather, a 34-year-old F.B.I. (Federal Bureau of Investigation) special agent, presented to her dentist with a "toothache." Examination of Heather's teeth including full mouth x-rays revealed no abnormality. Her dentist cleaned her teeth and discharged her. Now Heather informs you that she has had her "toothache" for 10 days. Her "toothache" is worse when she brushes her teeth and when she applies her makeup. She has no fever. There is no swelling of her teeth and jaws. She does not smoke. She is physically fit, vegetarian, with a known normal lipid profile.

   Your diagnosis is:

   A) An impacted wisdom tooth
   B) A jaw abscess
   C) Trigeminal neuralgia
   D) Acute anterior wall myocardial infarction
   E) None of the above

239. Which medication would you provide for Heather for her Tic Douloureux (trigeminal neuralgia)?

   A) Haloperidol (Haldol)
   B) Diazepam (Valium)
   C) Carbamazepine (Tegretol)
   D) Digoxin (Lanoxin)
   E) Metformin (Glucophage)

240. Bill a 27-year-old Family Practice Resident, corners you at a social gathering for physicians. Bill wants to know what you think is the cause of his unilateral facial paralysis. Bill has his 4-year-old daughter with him.

Your diagnosis is:

A) Osler-Weber-Rendu Disorder
B) Sturge-Weber-Dimitri Disorder
C) Ramsey-Hunt Disorder
D) All of the above
E) None of the above

241. Which of the following is the **MOST** probable etiology of Bill's unilateral facial palsy?

A) Varicella (chickenpox virus)
B) Malignancy
C) Spousal abuse
D) All of the above
E) None of the above

242. As Bill is leaving the social gathering he inquires, "What should I take?"

In addition to a complete examination, you recommend:

A) Zidovudine
B) Lamivudine
C) Indianavir
D) Acyclovir
E) Motrin

243. Sandra, a 37-year-old divorced associate professor of English, decided to begin exercising when her significant other, the offensive-line football coach, jokingly referred to her as "chubby," and after her department chair, a 52-year-old woman, successfully completed a 100-mile, week-end bike race. Sandra fell off of her bike striking her jaw on the concrete. In the emergency room, while treating her "road rash," she was seen to have weakness of her right arm.

Which of the following might be reasonably expected symptoms?

A) Neck pain
B) Headache
C) Photophobia
D) Paresthesias in the right arm
E) All of the above

244. Physical examination of Sandra reveals unequal pupils (anisocoria).

What is your **MOST** reasonable working diagnosis?

A) Brain tumor
B) Brain abscess
C) Multiple Sclerosis (M.S.)
D) Amyotrophic Lateral sclerosis (A.L.S.)
E) Traumatic Carotid Artery Dissection

245. Which cranial nerve is involved in Sandra's anisocoria? *unequal pupils*

A) III
B) VI
C) I
D) V
E) VII

246. Roger, a 40-year-old postal worker has been receiving workers' compensation for pain and post post-traumatic stress disorder following a a dog attack on his mail route. He has been out of the work force for one year and is now considered permanent and stationary by treating physician.

Which of the following is **TRUE** of suicide risk?

A) Patients receiving workers' compensation payments for pain have been shown to be at two to three times greater risk for suicide than the general population
B) Patients receiving workers' compensation for pain are at the same risk for suicide as the general population
C) Patients receiving workers' compensation for pain are at the same risk for suicide as the psychiatric population
D) Patients receiving workers' compensation for pain are at higher risk for suicide than the general psychiatric population
E) The potential for a future financial settlement has been shown to reduce the risk of suicide in chronic pain patients

247. Which of the following is true of chronic pain and post-traumatic stress disorder?

A) Systematic desensitization is relatively contraindicated in patients with chronic pain and post-traumatic stress disorder
B) About one thirds of individuals reporting headaches and related pain after a motor vehicle accident will meet the criteria for post traumatic stress disorder
C) Pain is not a common concomitant of post traumatic stress disorder
D) Psychological trauma is rarely a cause for delays in functional recovery
E) Post traumatic stress disorder is not associated with a significant impairment in functioning

248. Which are true of non-steroidal anti-inflammatories used in management of chronic pain:

A) Dyspepsia is a reliable predictor of ulceration
B) A one week trial is considered sufficiently adequate for benign pain syndromes
C) A three day trial is considered sufficiently adequate for malignant pain syndromes
D) NSAIDS are associated with hypernatremia
E) NSAIDS are associated with hyperkalemia

Medtext Medical World, Inc.

249.   Which of the following drugs is a mixed agonist-antagonist opioid:

    A) Buprenorphine
    B) Codeine
    C) Morphine
    D) Fentanyl
    E) Methadone

250.   Which of the following opiate drugs has the longest half-life:

    A) Morphine
    B) Hydromorphone
    C) Methadone
    D) Fentanyl
    E) Oxycodone

Single
Best
Answers

1. **B** **Social phobia describes the fear of embarrassing oneself in social situations while agoraphobia describes the fear of being unable to escape during a panic attack**

Social phobia is an anxiety disorder in which a person fears being in social or performance situations. The fear results from concerns of public embarrassment. Exposure to a social or performance situation leads to intense anxiety symptoms or even panic attacks. Panic disorder may be co-morbid. The presence of a companion often exacerbates social phobia. Effective treatments include antianxiety medication and behavioral therapies or a combination of the two. Agoraphobia, though often seen in combination with panic disorder, can occur without a diagnosis of panic disorder. Patients with this illness fear being in situations in which escape would be difficult if they were to experience panic symptoms or panic attacks. The fear is often alleviated by the presence of a companion. Treatment includes pharmacotherapy, behavioral therapy or a combination of the two.

1. Kaplan, HI, Saddock BJ (eds). Concise Textbook of Clinical Psychiatry, 7th edition. Williams and Wilkins, Baltimore, 1996:198, 204.

2. **D** **Obsessive Compulsive Disorder**

This patient appears to be in a disorganized psychotic state. Such a state can be induced by many psychiatric disorders. For example, substances, such as cocaine, often lead to manic like behavior and paranoia. Schizophrenia, disorganized subtype, is characterized by disorganized speech, disorganized behavior and flat or bizarre affect. Malingering, the intentional production of symptoms for secondary gain, could account for this behavior as well. Finally, culture bound syndromes, which describe locally specific patterns of bizarre behaviors, can cause this clinical picture. Amok, for example, is a syndrome originally reported in Malaysia. It consists of outbursts of violent, aggressive and disorganized behavior that appear to be self limited.

1. DSM IV TR, 4th edition. American Psychiatric Association, Washington, DC. 2000:244,315, 739, 898-899.

Medtext Medical World, Inc.

3.   A   Cataplexy

The diagnostic criteria for narcolepsy include refreshing REM sleep attacks, occurring daily for at least 3 months. Additional criteria include cataplexy (complete loss of muscle tone) and/or recurrent intrusions of REM sleep such as hypnagogic and hypnopompic hallucinations and sleep paralysis. Cataplexy is a common symptom seen in u p to 50% of cases.   Sleep paralysis, though included in the criteria for narcolepsy, is a rare symptom. It may also occur as isolated episodes in non-narcoleptic persons Increased job related accidents and a good response to stimulant medication are common, associated features of the illness, but are not necessary for a diagnosis.

1. Kaplan, HI, Saddock BJ (eds).   Concise Textbook of Clinical Psychiatry, 7th edition. Williams and Wilkins, Baltimore,1996:284.

4.   A   His age put him at an increased risk for attempting suicide compared with those younger than him

Approximately 95% of patients who attempt or commit suicide are thought to suffer from a psychiatric disorder, with depression accounting for 80%.   Studies have shown that depressed patients who have had violent suicides, such as by hanging, have lower levels of 5-HIAA levels in their cerebrospinal fluid than depressed patients who do not attempt suicide, or by depressed patients who die by less violent means. 53% of patients who suicide contact their physician in the month prior to attempting suicide and 80% contact their physician in the 6 months prior to suicide.   Physical illness is thought to contribute significantly to risk of suicide, especially if it is a chronic, disabling illness. The elderly attempt suicide less often than younger people but they complete suicide more often.

1. Kaplan, HI, Saddock BJ (eds).   Concise Textbook of Clinical Psychiatry, 7th edition.   Williams and Wilkins, Baltimore,1996: 361-366

Medtext Medical World, Inc.

5.   **A**   **Bipolar I, most recent episode manic, with mood incongruent hallucinations and delusions**

Criteria for a manic episode are met in this patient who has an irritable mood and at least 3 out of 7 associated symptoms including psychomotor agitation, increased risk taking behavior, and a decreased need for sleep. In order for this patient to be diagnosed with a mixed episode, she would simultaneously need to meet criteria for a Major Depressive Episode. Though not a criteria for diagnosis, mania is often accompanied by psychosis, which is often mood congruent. This patient, however, is having auditory hallucinations that are inconsistent with her mood state, or mood incongruent hallucinations.

1. Kaplan, HI, Saddock BJ (eds). Concise Textbook of Clinical Psychiatry, 7th edition. Williams and Wilkins, Baltimore MD. 1996:26,164.

6.   **B**   **Induce a major increase in a patient's weight**

Haloperidol, a typical neuroleptic, is more likely than olanzapine to cause extrapyramidal side effects (EPS) such as acute dystonic reactions. Patients predisposed to movement disorders, such as patients with underlying Parkinson's disease, are particularly sensitive to the EPS effects of typical neuroleptics. Olanzepine (Zyprexa), an atypical antipsychotic, is less likely to cause EPS in patients, but more likely to cause constipation than is haloperidol. This is likely due to the moderate anticholinergic effects of olanzepine. Though haloperidol has been known to precipitate some weight gain, weight gain a major side effect of the atypical agent olanzepine. In clinical trials, up to 40% of patients on olanzepine gain substantial weight on therapeutic doses. Both olanzepine and haloperidol can prolong the QT interval on EKG (electrocardiogram), though whether or not one agent is significantly more offensive than the other is not currently known.

1. Arana, George W., Rosenbaum F. Jerrold. Handbook of Psychiatric Drug Therapy, 4th Edition. Lippincott, Williams and Wilkins, Philadelphia PA. 2000:36-49.

Medtext Medical World, Inc.

7.   **C**   **Head CT without contrast**

In order to properly evaluate sleep disorders it is important to obtain a detailed history of the sleep wake complaint and its associated symptoms. A full psychiatric history must be obtained, and screens such as the Beck Depression Inventory can help in evaluating Axis I disorders such as major depression that could be contributing to the sleep disturbance. Interview with bed partners or tape recordings of sleep to assess for abnormal breathing can help in ruling out sleep apnea as a cause of the sleep disturbance. Polysomnography is a detailed lab based evaluation of sleep used to help in the diagnosis of insomnia and may include an EEG, EKG, O2 sat, evaluation of eye movements and measurement of muscle tone during sleep.

1. Jerald, Kay, Tasman, Allan and Lieberman, Jeffrey A. Psychiatry, Behavioral Science and Clinical Essentials. W.B. Saunders Company, Philadelphia PA. 2000: 460-461.

8.   **E**   **Exposing the patient to panic like somatic sensations by recreating the sensations during the session**

Interoceptive exposure is used often in the treatment of panic disorder. It involves having a patient deliberately hyperventilate or perform other actions that simulate the physiologic symptoms of a panic attack. The therapist then discourages avoidance behavior during the acts. Later in treatment, patients expose themselves to real life events that have induced panic symptoms in the past. A similar type of therapy, eye movement desensitization and reprocessing (EMDR) exposes patients to images and body sensations associated with panic while the patient tracks the therapist's finger with his/her eyes.

1. Kaplan, HI, Saddock BJ (eds). Comprehensive Textbook of Clinical Psychiatry, 7th edition. Lippincott, Williams and Wilkins, Philadelphia PA. 2000:2116-2117.

9. **B** **This patient's lithium dose should be decreased by half a couple of weeks prior to delivery**

Due to fluid shifts around the time of delivery and the potential for toxicity, patient's taking lithium should have their dose decreased by 50% in the two weeks prior to the date of confinement. Psychotropic medications are best avoided during the first trimester of pregnancy due to their teratogenic effects. During the second and third trimesters of pregnancy, risk of teratogenicity due to medications decreases, and the risks resulting from the psychiatric illness itself, in some patients, may outweigh the risks of the medications. The risk of neural tube defects from valproic acid during the first trimester of pregnancy is presently thought to be greater than the risk of teratogenicity from lithium during this same time period. Valproic acid is more efficacious than lithium in patients with mixed episodes.

1. Kaplan, HI, Saddock BJ (eds). Comprehensive Textbook of Clinical Psychiatry, 7th edition. Lippincott, Williams and Wilkins, Philadelphia PA. 2000:1950, 2384, 2290-2291.

10. **A** **A significant history of depression coexisting with the above symptoms would preclude a diagnosis of schizophrenia**

According to the DSM IV, schizoaffective disorder and mood disorders with psychotic features must be considered before diagnosing schizophrenia in a patient. Therefore, if mood episodes occur concurrently with active phase symptoms for a significant period of time, schizophrenia may not be diagnosed until the former two disorders are ruled out. Mood congruent delusions are more commonly seen in psychotic mood disorders, whereas bizarre delusions, such as transmitters implanted in one's head, are more reflective of schizophrenia. Approximately 10% of schizophrenic patients have a late onset in the fifth and sixth decades of life and these patients are more commonly women. A duration criterion for untreated schizophrenia is six months of symptoms including at least one month of active phase symptoms. Both schizophrenia and mood disorders can result in significant social and occupational dysfunction.

1. Kaplan, HI, Saddock BJ (eds). Comprehensive Textbook of Clinical Psychiatry, 7th edition. Lippincott, Williams and Wilkins, Philadelphia PA. 2000:1172, 1194-1195 3074-3075.

11.	E	**Brainstem stroke below the pons**
12.	A	**Intravenous rt-PA**
13.	A	**You would consider it appropriate therapy**
14.	E	**Sub arachnoid hemorrhage has occurred as a consequence of his stroke**
15.	A	**Delayed surgery**

This patient's history is quite consistent with cardioembolic stroke. Thrombotic strokes tend to occur during the early morning hours when hypercoagulability is at its peak. Embolic strokes are sudden, associated with severe deficits since there is no collateral circulation and on the CT scan reveal a wedge shaped infarct, often hemorrhagic, due to a re-flow phenomenon. Intracerebral hemorrhage is most often associated with headaches, more gradual progression of symptoms. If the patient survives, the chances of a good recovery are better than with ischemic strokes.

Patients with acute ischemic strokes seen within the first 3 hours should be considered for thrombolysis with intravenous rt-PA. Intra-arterial thrombolysis is not commonly possible because it requires an interventional radiologist and specialized instrumentation. However if available, it is superior to intravenous thrombolysis in ICA and large MCA stenosis. In this case in a small local hospital it is unlikely that an interventional ist or enough experience exists for safe intra-arterial therapy. Before attempting thrombolysis a number of conditions need to be excluded, labs including the blood sugar, platelets, PT, PTT and INR should be normal. Patients should not have hemorrhage on the head CT scan, nor should the early signs of infarction extend beyond 1/3 of the middle cerebral artery territory. With successful treatment patients have a 33% grater chance of being free of disability at 3 months compared to their counterparts who were not treated.

Thrombolysis caries a 6.6 % greater risk of intracranial hemorrhage (> 50% are fatal).

With a post rt-PA hemorrhage an urgent CT scan should be done. Platelets and cryoprecipitates should be administered and an urgent neurosurgical consultation obtained.

1. Moonis M et al. Cerebrovascular disease in Intensive Care Medicine, Irwin RS, Rippe JM(eds), Lippincott Williams and Wilkins, Baltimore MD. 2003:1885-1893.

16.   **B**   **Anterior cerebellar artery occlusion**

17.   **A**   **A single acute infarct in the lateral medullary region**

18.   **C**   **Hemiparesis**

19.   **C**   **Excellent**

20.   **A**   **Dysphagia**

Symptoms of vertigo, dysphagia, and dysarthria point to a brain stem lesion and are not compatible with an anterior cerebral artery syndrome. Lateral medullary syndrome is secondary to infarction of the lateral medulla and the signs associated with it include crossed sensory loss to pain and temperature over the ipsilateral face and contralateral limbs. This is associated with dysphagia, vertigo, dysarthria and an ipsilateral Horner syndrome. The usual cause is thrombosis of the ipsilateral vertebral artery and less commonly occlusion of the posterior inferior cerebral artery.

1. Adams RD, Victor M, Roper AH. Cerebrovascular diseases in Principles of Neurology, 6th Edition. McGraw Hill, New York NY. 1997:831-832.

21.   **C**   **REM behavior disorder**

22.   **C**   **Rolandic epilepsy**

23.   **A**   **Frontal lobe epilepsy**

24.   **A**   **Polysomnogram**

25.   **D**   **Clonazepam (Klonopin)**

Rapid Eye movement (REM) behavior disorder is not uncommon in the elderly population and is especially prominent in patients with dementia, Parkinson disease, multisystem degeneration and patients on certain antidepressants. The manifestations are violent enactment of dreams often leading to injury to the bed partner. Pathophysiologically there is loss of motor inhibition that is normally present during REM sleep. Clonazepam (Klonapin) is effective in suppressing REM behavior disorder related nocturnal attacks.

1. Kryger MH, Roth T, Dement WC. Principles and practice of sleep medicine, 3rd Edition. WB Saunders Company, Philadelphia PA. 2000:724-742.

Medtext Medical World, Inc.

26.	B	3RD Nerve (fascicular)
27.	D	Ischemic neuropathy
28.	D	Chest CT scan
29.	B	Good
30.	A	Low

This patient had an acute onset of a third nerve palsy with sparing of the pupils. This is an important difference between compressive third nerve lesions as in herniation, aneurysmal compression, tumors etc., and ischemic third nerve lesions that spare the pupillary fibers. This is not an absolute rule and if compressive lesions are suspected from the history, an imaging study is appropriate. The commonest cause of an ischemic third nerve lesion is diabetes but it can also be seen in vasculitis, paraproteinemias (where the ESR may be very high) and in temporal arteritis. Recovery is the rule and most patients tend to make a complete recovery in 1-4 months. Patients with well controlled diabetes are at a very low risk of recurrence.

1. Adams RD, Victor M, Roper AH. Cerebrovascular diseases in Principles of Neurology, 6th Edition. McGraw Hill, New York NY. 1997:777-873.

31. **A** **Detailed history and examination**

32. **E** **All of the above are possibilities**

Loss of sensations in the legs with areflexia
Resting tremors of the upper extremities
No findings
Conjunctival pallor

33. **A** **Polysomnogram**

34. **E** **A and B**

Sleep fragmentation
Periodic leg movements of sleep

35. **A** **Low serum ferritin**

A number of sleep related conditions can lead to excessive daytime sleepiness and fatigue. The common conditions are insomnia, sleep fragmentation because of obstructive apneas, hypopneas or upper airway resistance syndrome, periodic leg movements of sleep often but not invariably associated with restless leg movements and narcolepsy. The history differs. It is important to get as accurate a history from the patient and the bed partner. The latter is valuable in documenting if the patient has abnormal snoring, thrashing about (PLMS), recurrent arousals etc. This should be the first step in diagnosis. An all night polysomnogram would reveal if there are obstructive sleep apnea associated with desaturations and arousals, PLMS associated with arousals and sleep fragmentation etc. MSLT is indicated if the PSG cannot explain the symptoms or in suspected narcolepsy.

This patient's history is very suggestive of restless leg syndrome and the PSG is likely to show PLMS with arousals and sleep fragmentation. RLS can be secondary to iron deficiency anemia, peripheral neuropathy, medications and extrapyramidal disorders.

Therefore patients should be investigated for the same. The most effective treatment is with Levodopa (Sinemet) or dopamine agonists given in low doses at night. Other options include clonazepam (Klonopin), gabapentin (Neurontin) and opioids. If a reversible cause is found it should be effectively treated.

1. Kryger MH, Roth T, Dement WC. Principles and practice of sleep medicine, 3rd Edition. WB Saunders Company, Philadelphia PA. 2000:742-752.

36.   **C**   **Midline brain tumor**

37.   **A**   **Early dementia**

38.   **E**   **Cortical atrophy alone**

39.   **D**   **Clinical response to removal of 30 cc of CSF**

40.   **E**   **Cortical atrophy alone**

NPH is a common condition and in the vast majority not symptomatic, and should not be treated. The usual clinical presentation is with early gait disturbances from compression of the descending white matter tracts, incontinence, resulting from the same mechanism and dementia which includes memory loss as well as frontal lobe dysfunction. A CT or MRI shows ventriculomegaly with rounding of the frontal horns, and this ventriculomegaly is out of proportion to any cortical atrophy. This is important, since loss of brain volume itself causes ventricular enlargement, an ex-vacuo effect. However if early incontinence and ataxia followed by dementia are seen, an attempt should be made to see if shunting would be helpful in reversing symptoms. The most predictive test is removal of large quantities of CSF and observes any improvement in symptoms. Radioisotope studies are helpful in making the diagnosis but do not consistently predict a therapeutic response. Patients with early dementia without the other features are unlikely to have NPH and unless a clear clinical response to the lumbar puncture is seen, shunting should not be attempted.

1. Adams RD, Victor M, Roper AH. Principles of Neurology, 6th Edition. McGraw Hill, New York NY. 1997:634-638.

41.   **E**   Occipital involving bilateral occipital poles

42.   **E**   Retinitis pigmentosa

43.   **E**   Multiple sclerosis

44.   **E**   Migraine with aura

45.   **E**   Muscle contraction headaches

Causes of visual loss in a patient with history of migraine headaches may be because of complicated migraine, vasoconstrictors used to treat migraine, concomitant use of oral contraceptive pill, mitochondrial disorders with migraine like headaches. In this case, the medications were given to a patient with hypertension and migraine. Hypertension is a contraindication to use of vasoconstrictors and probably led to the visual loss.

1. Laskowitz D, et al. Acute visual loss and other disturbances of the eyes in Neurologic clinics (neurological emergencies) Feske SK and Wen PY (Eds),1998:323-353.

46.   **E**   Nerve conduction studies

47.   **C**   CADASIL

48.   **C**   Anticardiolipin antibody syndrome

49.   **B**   Low dose aspirin

50.   **D**   Heparin

Migraine with aura is a risk factor for stroke. The antiphospholipid antibody syndrome comprises of history of recurrent fetal loss, thrombocytopenia, migraine, stroke and presence of anticardiolipin antibodies. The PTT is prolonged and remains uncorrected with mixing the blood with normal blood. Triptans are contraindicated with hypertension, heart disease, basilar and hemiplegic migraine but not in migraine with aura.

1. Headache in Clinical Practice Silberstein SD, Lipton RB and Goadsby PJ (Eds):ISIS Medical Media 1998:61-90.

Medtext Medical World, Inc.

51.	E	Occipital lobe
52.	E	Neuropsychiatric intervention
53.	E	Transient ischemic attack
54.	B	Admit for a detailed workup
55.	C	5% develop a stroke within 2 days

Patients may appear to be confused because of many reasons. Toxic-metabolic encephalopathy, transient global amnesia, following head trauma, following or during non-convulsive seizures, with confusional migraine and stroke affecting the Wernicke area. This latter possibility should always be considered in patients presenting with fluent aphasia as is the case here. The common practice of discharging patients home after a TIA is to be condemned as 10.5 % have a stroke within 30 days and 50% of these occur in the first 48 hours. Patients should be admitted and a full stroke work-up and appropriate management instituted.

1. Johnson et al. JAMA 2000:2901.

56.	E	Migraine with aura
57.	A	Tumor
58.	D	Evoked potentials (visual and somatosensory)
59.	D	High dose steroids
60.	A	Meningitis

Patients presenting with rapid visual loss associated with headaches point to several etiologies including central retinal artery embolism, temporal arteritis, multiple sclerosis, cavernous sinus thrombosis (usually patient is very sick with meningismus and high grade fever, with a prior history of a pustule in the dangerous area of the face), mitochondrial disorders such as MELAS, Leber's disease, subarachnoid hemorrhage secondary to rupture of an ophthalmic artery aneurysm. In cases of temporal arteritis there is headache, temporal artery tenderness and reduced pulsations and elevated liver enzymes with or without EKG changes. Because of skip lesions a temporal artery biopsy may be negative

Medtext Medical World, Inc.

(wise to get bilateral biopsies). Visual loss can be very rapid and steroids should be initiated immediately without waiting for a biopsy. The dose of long term steroids should be the minimum required to abolish symptoms and normalize the ESR. Long term therapy is the rule as the disease may run its course up to 2 years. If patients are steroid intolerant or run the risk of complications, chemotherapeutic agents may be instituted as a steroid sparing strategy.

1. Headache in Clinical Practice Silberstein SD, Lipton RB and Goadsby PJ (Eds):ISIS Medical Media 1998:61-90.

61.   **D**   **Specific phobia because she is afraid of dogs**

Specific phobia is an irrational fear of certain situations or objects (e.g., animals, heights, needles). The patient avoids the feared situation or object. Specific phobia has a lifetime prevalence of 7-11% in the population. There is no effective pharmacologic treatment for specific phobias. Systematic desensitization with reciprocal inhibition is most effective. Short-term benzodiazepines and beta-blockers to control autonomic symptoms may help during sensitization.

1. Fadem,B., Simring, S. High Yield Psychiatry. 2nd Edition. Lippincott, Williams & Wilkins, Philadelphia PA. 2003:77.

2. Kaplan, HI., Sadock BJ. A Comprehensive Textbook of Psychiatry. Williams & Wilkins, Baltimore MD. 1999:1441-1503.

62.   **A**   **Obsessive compulsive disorder**

Patients with obsessive compulsive disorder (OCD) experience recurring intrusive feelings, thoughts, and images (obsessions) which cause anxiety. The anxiety is relieved in part by performing repetitive actions (compulsions). Common obsessions and compulsions include contamination, checking, counting, and putting things in order. Patients usually realize that these thoughts and behaviors are irrational and want to eliminate them. OCD is associated with other anxiety disorders, major depressive disorder, obsessive compulsive personality disorder, eating disorders, and Tourette disorder.

1. Kaplan, HI., Sadock BJ. A Comprehensive Textbook of Psychiatry. Williams & Wilkins, Baltimore MD. 1999:1441-1503.

63.   **D**   **OCD symptoms may first appear following a significant life stressor**

Psychosocial factors may be involved as symptoms of OCD often first appear after a stressful life experience. It is equally common in women and men and occurs in 2-3% of the population. It usually starts in childhood or young adulthood. Genetic factors likely play a role as the concordance rate is increased in first degree relatives of patients with OCD and is higher in monozygotic than in dizygotic twins. In one-third of patients, symptoms improve significantly with treatment; in one-half, symptoms improve moderately; in the rest, symptoms do not improve or progressive deterioration in functioning occurs. Patients often have insight into their condition and seek to eliminate or minimize their symptoms.

1. Fadem,B., Simring, S. High Yield Psychiatry. 2nd Edition. Lippincott, Williams & Wilkins, Philadelphia PA. 2003:78.

2. Kaplan, HI., Sadock BJ. A Comprehensive Textbook of Psychiatry. Williams & Wilkins, Baltimore MD. 1999:1441-1503.

64.   **C**   **Generalized anxiety disorder**

Patients with generalized anxiety disorder (GAD) have persistent symptoms of anxiety, including hyperarousal that lasts at least 6 months. The symptoms of anxiety in GAD are unrelated to a specific person or situation (free-floating anxiety). Approximately one-half of patients with GAD have chronic symptoms which wax and wane and require treatment indefinitely. GAD is slightly more common in women with a lifetime prevalence of 5%. In 50% of patients, onset occurs during childhood or adolescence.

1. Fadem,B., Simring, S. High Yield Psychiatry. 2nd Edition. Lippincott, Williams & Wilkins, Philadelphia PA. 2003:79.

2. Kaplan, HI., Sadock BJ. A Comprehensive Textbook of Psychiatry. Williams & Wilkins, Baltimore MD. 1999:1441-1503.

Medtext Medical World, Inc.

65.   **B**   **Post traumatic stress disorder (PTSD)**

Post traumatic stress disorder (PTSD) occurs when a catastrophic event (usually life-threatening or potentially fatal, e.g., war, terrorist attack, earthquake, serious accident, robbery) affects the patient or a close friend or relative. PTSD patients experience both hyperarousal (anxiety, nightmares, hypervigilance) and withdrawal (survivor guilt, dissociation, social withdrawal). Symptoms must last for at least one month. Symptoms lasting 2 days to 4 weeks following a catastrophic event are diagnosed as acute stress disorder. If the catastrophic event is not life threatening (bankruptcy, divorce) the symptoms would indicate an adjustment disorder.

1. Fadem,B., Simring, S. High Yield Psychiatry. 2nd Edition. Lippincott, Williams & Wilkins, Philadelphia PA. 2003:79.

2. Kaplan, HI., Sadock BJ. A Comprehensive Textbook of Psychiatry. Williams & Wilkins, Baltimore MD. 1999:1441-1503.

66.   **E**   **Up to half of victims of catastrophic events will meet criteria for PTSD**

Post traumatic stress disorder (PTSD) occurs when a catastrophic event (usually life-threatening or potentially fatal) affects the patient or a close friend or relative. The lifetime prevalence of PTSD is 8%. 50% of patients recover completely within 3 months. Group therapy must be initiated as soon as possible after the traumatic event. Some limited success with antidepressants (SSRIs), anticonvulsants (flashbacks and nightmares), and beta-blockers for control of autonomic symptoms.

1. Fadem,B., Simring, S. High Yield Psychiatry. 2nd Edition. Lippincott, Williams & Wilkins, Philadelphia PA. 2003:79.

2. Kaplan, HI., Sadock BJ. A Comprehensive Textbook of Psychiatry. Williams & Wilkins, Baltimore MD. 1999:1441-1503.

67.   **A**   **Somatization disorder**

Somatoform disorders (such as somatization disorder) are characterized by physical symptoms without a sufficient organic cause. A person who has somatoform disorder is not faking and not delusional, but truly believes he has a physical problem. The most important differential diagnosis of the somatoform disorders is unidentified organic disease. The characteristics of somatization disorder include a history of multiple somatic complaints over many years, including: 4 pain symptoms (e.g., headache), 2 gastrointestinal symptoms (e.g. nausea), 1 sexual symptom (e.g., menstrual irregularities), 1 pseudoneurological symptom (e.g., paralysis). These chronic and lifelong symptoms are increased by stressful life events.

1. Fadem,B., Simring, S. High Yield Psychiatry. 2nd Edition. Lippincott, Williams & Wilkins, Philadelphia PA. 2003:82-84.

2. Kaplan, HI., Sadock BJ. A Comprehensive Textbook of Psychiatry. Williams & Wilkins, Baltimore MD. 1999:1504-1544.

68.   **A**   **Conversion disorder**

Conversion disorder is marked by the abrupt, dramatic loss of motor or sensory function, often with an obvious or symbolic significance. The most common motor symptoms are paralysis with absent pathologic reflexes, bizarre seizures, and globus hystericus (lump in the throat). The most common sensory presentations are paresthesias, anesthesias (often inconsistent with anatomic innervation), and visual problems with normal evoked potentials. Conversion disorder is more common in psychiatrically unsophisticated patients and comorbid with histrionic personality disorder. Symptoms often remit in less than one month. Symptoms may recur in up to one fourth of patients during stressful life events.

1. Fadem,B., Simring, S. High Yield Psychiatry. 2nd Edition. Lippincott, Williams & Wilkins, Philadelphia PA. 2003:81-84.

2. Kaplan, HI., Sadock BJ. A Comprehensive Textbook of Psychiatry. Williams & Wilkins, Baltimore MD. 1999:1504-1544.

69. **E** **Hypochondriasis**

Hypochondriasis is a somatoform disorder. Hypochondriasis is marked by exaggerated concern with health and illness over at least a 6 month period that continues despite medical evaluation and reassurance by a physician. It is more common in middle and old age. Symptoms may last for as long as a few years; these periods alternate with periods when few symptoms are present. As many as 50% of patients improve over the course of their lives.

1. Fadem,B., Simring, S. High Yield Psychiatry. 2nd Edition. Lippincott, Williams & Wilkins, Philadelphia PA. 2003:82-83.

2. Kaplan, HI., Sadock BJ. A Comprehensive Textbook of Psychiatry. Williams & Wilkins, Baltimore MD. 1999:1504-1544.

70. **B** *Body dysmorphic disorder*

Body dysmorphic disorder is a somatoform disorder. Body dysmorphic disorder is the excessive focus on a minor or imagined physical defect (usually of the face or head). Onset of the disorder usually occurs in the late teens. Level of concern varies over time. Plastic surgery or medical treatment must be used conservatively as it rarely relieves the symptoms.

1. Fadem,B., Simring, S. High Yield Psychiatry. 2nd Edition. Lippincott, Williams & Wilkins, Philadelphia PA. 2003:82-83.

2. Kaplan, HI., Sadock BJ. A Comprehensive Textbook of Psychiatry. Williams & Wilkins, Baltimore MD. 1999:1504-1544.

Medtext Medical World, Inc.

71. **B** **Pain disorder**

Pain disorder is a protracted, intense discomfort not explained adequately by physical causes. It can be acute or chronic and often coexists with a medical condition. Onset of the disorder is usually in the thirties or forties. It can be disabling, particularly if there is a significant physiological component to the patient's symptoms. The patient may become dependent on pain medications. Antidepressants with serotonin activity may be beneficial.

1. Fadem,B., Simring, S. High Yield Psychiatry. 2nd Edition. Lippincott, Williams & Wilkins, Philadelphia PA. 2003:82-83.

2. Kaplan, HI., Sadock BJ. A Comprehensive Textbook of Psychiatry. Williams & Wilkins, Baltimore MD. 1999:1441-1503.

72. **A** **Factitious disorder by proxy**

In contrast to patients with somatoform disorders (who truly believe that they are ill), patients with factitious disorder know that they are pretending to have a mental or physical illness or actually inducing physical illness to obtain medical attention. In factitious disorder by proxy, an adult, usually a parent feigns or induces illness in a child to obtain medical attention. Factitious disorder by proxy is a form of child abuse and must be reported to child welfare authorities.

1. Fadem,B., Simring, S. High Yield Psychiatry. 2nd Edition. Lippincott, Williams & Wilkins, Philadelphia PA. 2003:84.

2. Kaplan, HI., Sadock BJ. A Comprehensive Textbook of Psychiatry. Williams & Wilkins, Baltimore MD. 1999:1533-1543.

73.   A   Malingering

Malingering is the conscious simulation or exaggeration of physical or mental illness for financial or other obvious gains (e.g., avoiding work or incarceration). In contrast to the patient with factitious disorder who seeks medical treatment, the malingering patient avoids treatment. Symptoms often improve after the patient obtains the desired gain. Malingering may be more common in men than in women. It is often seen in adults with antisocial personality disorder and in children and adolescents with conduct disorder.

1. Fadem,B., Simring, S. High Yield Psychiatry. 2nd Edition. Lippincott, Williams & Wilkins, Philadelphia PA. 2003:84.

2. Kaplan, HI., Sadock BJ. A Comprehensive Textbook of Psychiatry. Williams & Wilkins, Baltimore MD. 1999:1433-1443.

74.   B   Dissociative amnesia

Dissociative amnesia is characterized by an inability to recall important data about oneself. It usually affects young adults and women and is relatively uncommon. The etiology of dissociative amnesia is the use of the defense mechanisms of repression and denial after a recent emotionally traumatic event. Treatment includes hypnosis and sodium amobarbital interview to recover traumatic memories and long-term psychotherapy to deal with the recovered material. Amnesia after acute stress usually resolves in minutes or days, occasionally lasts for years.

1. Fadem,B., Simring, S. High Yield Psychiatry. 2nd Edition. Lippincott, Williams & Wilkins, Philadelphia PA. 2003:86.

2. Kaplan, HI., Sadock BJ. A Comprehensive Textbook of Psychiatry. Williams & Wilkins, Baltimore MD. 1999:1544-1576.

Medtext Medical World, Inc.

75. **E** **All of the above**

Substance abuse
Head injury
Delirium
Seizure disorder

Dissociative disorders are characterized by sudden but temporary loss of memory or identity or by feelings of detachment because of emotional factors. The medical differential diagnosis for dissociative disorders includes: substance abuse, head injury, sequelae of electroconvulsive therapy (ECT) or anesthesia, seizure disorder, delirium, and dementia. The psychological differential diagnosis of the dissociative disorders includes post-traumatic stress disorder (PTSD) and malingering. Members of some religions or cultures view altered states of perception, identity, or consciousness in the framework of particular experiences such as a trance state entered into at a religious revival meeting. In these frameworks, dissociation may not be abnormal.

1. Fadem,B., Simring, S. High Yield Psychiatry. 2nd Edition. Lippincott, Williams & Wilkins, Philadelphia PA. 2003:85.

2. Kaplan, HI., Sadock BJ. A Comprehensive Textbook of Psychiatry. Williams & Wilkins, Baltimore MD. 1999:1544-1576.

76. **B** **Psychogenic fugue**

Dissociation occurs when the individual deals with emotional conflict or internal or external stressors with a breakdown in the usually integrated functions or consciousness, memory, perception of self or the environment, or sensory/motor behavior. Dissociative fugue or psychogenic fugue is characterized by the sudden inability to remember pertinent personal information coupled with leaving home, moving away, and taking on a different identity. The person is usually not aware that she has assumed a new identity. The disorder is rare. It is associated with a history of excessive alcohol use.

1. Fadem,B., Simring, S. High Yield Psychiatry. 2nd Edition. Lippincott, Williams & Wilkins, Philadelphia PA. 2003:87.

2. Kaplan, HI., Sadock BJ. A Comprehensive Textbook of Psychiatry. Williams & Wilkins, Baltimore MD. 1999:1544-1577.

77.   **B**   **Dissociative identity disorder**

Dissociative identity disorder is characterized by at least two separate personalities or "alters" within one individual. Patients often have five to ten alters, or more. Most patients are women (although some of the alters may be male), and one personality usually dominates the others. Mild forms of dissociative identity disorder may resemble borderline personality disorder or schizophrenia. When the patient presents in a legal or forensic setting (person in jail for a crime they cannot remember), malingering and alcohol abuse must be excluded.

1. Fadem,B., Simring, S. High Yield Psychiatry. 2nd Edition. Lippincott, Williams & Wilkins, Philadelphia PA. 2003:87.

2. Kaplan, HI., Sadock BJ. A Comprehensive Textbook of Psychiatry. Williams & Wilkins, Baltimore MD. 1999:1544-1576.

78.   **A**   **Depersonalization disorder**

Depersonalization disorder is characterized by recurrent and persistent feelings of detachment from the self, social situation, or environment (derealization). Symptoms of depersonalization and derealization often occur in patients with other psychiatric disorders, such as schizophrenia, depression, anxiety, and histrionic and borderline personality disorder. The patient has normal reality testing. Depersonalization causes clinically significant distress or impairment in social, occupational, or other important areas of functioning. Mild symptoms may occur in normal people when they are exposed to an unfamiliar environment or when they are under the stress of a physical or psychological trauma.

1. Fadem,B., Simring, S. High Yield Psychiatry. 2nd Edition. Lippincott, Williams & Wilkins, Philadelphia PA. 2003:87.

2. Kaplan, HI., Sadock BJ. A Comprehensive Textbook of Psychiatry. Williams & Wilkins, Baltimore MD. 1999:1544-1576.

Medtext Medical World, Inc.

79.   **B**   **Dyspareunia**

Sexual dysfunction involves difficulty with an aspect of the sexual response cycle without an identifiable biological basis. The sexual pain disorders are dyspareunia and vaginismus. Dyspareunia is persistent pain associated with sexual intercourse. Dyspareunia is present in 3% of men and 15% of women of ages 18 to 59 years. Increasingly, primary care physicians are treating patients with sexual problems instead of referring them to sex therapists.

1. Fadem,B., Simring, S. High Yield Psychiatry. 2nd Edition. Lippincott, Williams & Wilkins, Philadelphia PA. 2003:91.

2. Kaplan, HI., Sadock BJ. A Comprehensive Textbook of Psychiatry. Williams & Wilkins, Baltimore MD. 1999:1577-1662.

80.   **B**   **Vaginismus**

Vaginismus is characterized by painful spasm of the outer one-third of the vagina. It is uncommon in clinical practice. Treatments for sexual dysfunction include: sex therapy; behavioral therapy and relaxation techniques, including hypnosis; self-stimulation; pharmacological and surgical techniques. The treatment of comorbid drug and alcohol abuse should be undertaken. Patients who have serious relationship problems or a history of sexual abuse or rape may benefit from marital counseling and dual sex therapy (a male and a female therapist see the couple together).

1. Fadem,B., Simring, S. High Yield Psychiatry. 2nd Edition. Lippincott, Williams & Wilkins, Philadelphia PA. 2003:91.

2. Kaplan, HI., Sadock BJ. A Comprehensive Textbook of Psychiatry.Williams & Wilkins, Baltimore MD. 1999:1577-1662.

81.   **A**   **Premature ejaculation**

Stages of the sexual response cycle include excitement, plateau, orgasm and resolution. Premature ejaculation is characterized as ejaculation (orgasm) before the man would like it to occur. A short or absent plateau phase of the sexual response cycle is often associated with anxiety. Behavioral treatment techniques include the squeeze technique. With the squeeze technique, the man is taught to identify the sensation that occurs just before the emission phase, when he can no longer prevent ejaculation. At this moment, the man asks his partner to exert pressure on the coronal ridge of the glans on both sides of the penis until the erection subsides. Pharmacological treatments include selective serotonin reuptake inhibitors (SSRIs) to treat premature ejaculation because they delay orgasm.

1. Fadem,B., Simring, S. High Yield Psychiatry. 2nd Edition. Lippincott, Williams & Wilkins, Philadelphia PA. 2003:90.

2. Kaplan, HI., Sadock BJ. A Comprehensive Textbook of Psychiatry. Williams & Wilkins, Baltimore MD. 1999:1577-1662.

82.   D   Orgasmic disorder

There are two forms of orgasmic disorder: lifelong and acquired. Lifelong orgasmic disorder is described as the patient having had no previous orgasm. Acquired orgasmic disorder is the current inability to achieve orgasm despite adequate genital stimulation in the setting of normal orgasms in the past. The prevalence estimate for ages 18 to 59 years is 10% for men and 25% for women. The two most common female sexual dysfunction disorders are orgasmic disorder and hypoactive sexual desire disorder.

1. Fadem,B., Simring, S. High Yield Psychiatry. 2nd Edition. Lippincott, Williams & Wilkins, Philadelphia PA. 2003:90.

2. Kaplan, HI., Sadock BJ. A Comprehensive Textbook of Psychiatry. Williams & Wilkins, Baltimore MD. 1999:1577-1662.

83.   E   Impotence

Male erectile disorder (impotence) is found in three common variants: 1) primary or lifelong (rare) in which the man has never had an erection sufficient for penetration; 2) secondary or acquired (common) in which the man has current inability to maintain erections despite normal erections in the past; and 3) situational (common) in which the man has difficulty maintaining erections in some situations (with a partner), but not others (alone). The

Medtext Medical World, Inc.

prevalence estimate in people age 18 to 59 is 10%. Sildenafil (Viagra) is an effective agent for treating male erectile disorder. It works by increasing the availability of cGMP, a vasodilator that helps maintain penile erection, when a man is sexually stimulated. Systemic administration of opioid antagonists (e.g. naltrexone) or systemic (e.g. yohimbine) or intracorporeal administration of vasodilators (e.g. papaverine, phentolamine) may be used to treat erectile dysfunction. Implantation of a prosthetic device is a surgical treatment for male erectile disorder.

1. Fadem,B., Simring, S. High Yield Psychiatry. 2nd Edition. Lippincott, Williams & Wilkins, Philadelphia PA. 2003:90.

2. Kaplan, HI., Sadock BJ. A Comprehensive Textbook of Psychiatry. Williams & Wilkins, Baltimore MD. 1999:1577-1663.

84. B Female sexual arousal disorder

Female sexual arousal disorder has an estimated prevalence of 20% in the 18 to 59 years age group. It is characterized by the inability to maintain vaginal lubrication until the sex act is completed. This occurs despite adequate physical stimulation. Psychological etiologies include: current relationship problems, long-term psychological problems, incompatible sexual technique between partners, and fear and anxiety. Fear and anxiety may stem from: unconscious factors, performance anxiety, fear of pregnancy or commitment, fear of rejection or loss of control.

1. Fadem,B., Simring, S. High Yield Psychiatry. 2nd Edition. Lippincott, Williams & Wilkins, Philadelphia PA. 2003:90.

2. Kaplan, HI., Sadock BJ. A Comprehensive Textbook of Psychiatry. Williams & Wilkins, Baltimore MD. 1999:1577-1662.

85. B Sexual aversion disorder

Sexual aversion disorder is a sexual desire disorder. The disorder is characterized by aversion to and avoidance of sexual activity. The differential diagnosis of sexual disorders includes: unidentified general medical condition, side effects of medication, substance use or substance abuse, and alterations in the levels of the gonadal hormones. Androgen is the major sexual interest (libido) hormone in both men and women. Androgen is secreted by the adrenal glands as well as the gonads throughout adult life.

1. Fadem,B., Simring, S. High Yield Psychiatry. 2nd Edition. Lippincott, Williams & Wilkins, Philadelphia PA. 2003:90.

2. Kaplan, HI., Sadock BJ. A Comprehensive Textbook of Psychiatry. Williams & Wilkins, Baltimore MD. 1999:1577-1662.1577-1662.

86.　　A　Hypoactive sexual desire

Hypoactive sexual desire is a sexual desire disorder. It is a disorder of the excitement phase of the sexual response cycle. It is characterized by decreased interest in sexual activity. It may be normal individual variation in desire. Hypoactive sexual desire disorder and orgasmic disorder are the most common female sexual dysfunction disorders.

1. Fadem,B., Simring, S. High Yield Psychiatry. 2nd Edition. Lippincott, Williams & Wilkins, Philadelphia PA. 2003:90.

2. Kaplan, HI., Sadock BJ. A Comprehensive Textbook of Psychiatry. Williams & Wilkins, Baltimore MD. 1999:1577-1662.

87.　　B　Progesterone decreases sexual desire in both men and women

Estrogen is only minimally involved in sexual response in women; therefore, menopause and aging do not per se decrease sex drive in women. Estrogen may reduce sexual interest and behavior in men. Progesterone may inhibit sexual interest and behavior in women (contained in many birth control pill and hormone replacement preparations) and in men (used to treat prostate cancer and hypersexual conditions). Androgens are the major sexual interest (libido) hormone in both women and men. Androgen levels in men may be reduced by stress.

1. Fadem,B., Simring, S. High Yield Psychiatry. 2nd Edition. Lippincott, Williams & Wilkins, Philadelphia PA. 2003:91.

2. Kaplan, HI., Sadock BJ. A Comprehensive Textbook of Psychiatry. Williams & Wilkins, Baltimore MD. 1999:1577-1663.

88.   **C**   **Prenatal etiology for gender identity disorder has been suggested**

Gender identity disorder is commonly called trans-sexuality and is a person's subjective feeling that he has been born the wrong sex despite normal physiology; the person may take sex hormones or seek sex change surgery. The differential diagnosis of gender disorder includes physiological hermaphroditism, schizophrenia, and persistent and marked distress about one's own sexual orientation (sexual disorder, not otherwise specified). Gender identity disorder is more common in men and can often be diagnosed in childhood. The etiology is not known, but it may be associated with abnormal prenatal levels of sex hormones. Supportive psychotherapy is useful; however gender identity disorder is often associated with lifelong distress, depression and increased risk of suicide.

1. Fadem,B., Simring, S. High Yield Psychiatry. 2nd Edition. Lippincott, Williams & Wilkins, Philadelphia PA. 2003:95.

2. Kaplan, HI., Sadock BJ. A Comprehensive Textbook of Psychiatry. Williams & Wilkins, Baltimore MD. 1999:1577-1662.

89.   **B**   **Is a normal variant of sexual expression**

Homosexuality (e.g. having a gay or lesbian sexual orientation) is not considered a dysfunction in the DSM-IV-TR. Homosexuality is a normal variant of sexual expression. Distress about one's sexual preference is considered a dysfunction and now diagnosed as sexual disorder, not otherwise specified. Most gay or lesbian people have experienced heterosexual sex and many have had children. Homosexuality occurs in 3-10% of men and 1%-5% of women but may be underreported. No significant ethnic differences are seen. Genetic factors and alterations in prenatal hormone levels have been suggested as potential etiologies.

1. Fadem,B., Simring, S. High Yield Psychiatry. 2nd Edition. Lippincott, Williams & Wilkins, Philadelphia PA. 2003:96.

2. Kaplan, HI., Sadock BJ. A Comprehensive Textbook of Psychiatry. Williams & Wilkins, Baltimore MD. 1999:1577-1662.

90.   **A**   **Anorexia nervosa**

The psychological characteristics of anorexia nervosa include excessive dieting because of an overwhelming fear of being obese; refusal to eat despite normal appetite; abnormal behavior dealing with food; conflicts about sexuality; lack of interest in sex; "perfect child" syndrome; intrafamilial conflicts. The physical characteristics include weight loss (15% or more of normal body weight); amenorrhea (3 or more consecutive missed menstrual periods); metabolic acidosis; hypercholesterolemia; mild anemia; lanugo; melanosis coli. Anorexia nervosa occurs in about 0.5% of women. It is ten times more common in women than in men. Because starvation can lead to death, the goal of initial treatment is to restore the patient's nutritional status. If the patient's body weight decreases to 20% or more below normal, she may be admitted to the hospital and treated until she achieves near-normal body weight.

1. Fadem,B., Simring, S. High Yield Psychiatry. 2nd Edition. Lippincott, Williams & Wilkins, Philadelphia PA. 2003:99.

2. Kaplan, HI., Sadock BJ. A Comprehensive Textbook of Psychiatry. Williams & Wilkins, Baltimore MD. 1999:1577-1662.

91.   **C**   **Bulimia**

The psychological characteristics of bulimia are marked by binge eating (in secret) of high-calorie foods usually followed by vomiting or other purging behavior to avoid weight gain (binge eating and purging also occurs in some patients with anorexia nervosa); poor self image; serious concern about gaining weight; distress over the binge eating. Physical characteristics of bulimia include: relatively normal body weight; esophageal varices caused by repeated vomiting; enamel erosion especially in anterior teeth due to dental caries caused by gastric acid in the mouth; swelling or infection of the parotid glands; scars and/or calluses on the dorsal surfaces of the hand from the teeth because the hand is used to induce gagging; electrolyte disturbances; menstrual irregularities. Pharmacological treatment includes average to high doses of antidepressants, such as heterocyclics, selective serotonin reuptake inhibitors, and monoamine oxidase inhibitors. Combinations of cognitive therapy and antidepressants are most effective, even in the absence of depressive symptoms.

1. Fadem,B., Simring, S. High Yield Psychiatry. 2nd Edition. Lippincott, Williams & Wilkins, Philadelphia PA. 2003:99.

2. Kaplan, HI., Sadock BJ. A Comprehensive Textbook of Psychiatry. Williams & Wilkins, Baltimore MD. 1999:1663-1676.

92.   D   Kleptomania

Patients with impulse control disorders are unable to resist engaging in behavior that is harmful to themselves or other people. Patients usually experience increased tension before the behavior and relief or pleasure after the behavior is completed. Kleptomania is an impulse control disorder where the impulse is to take items without paying for them (even if they are affordable). The desire is taking, rather than owning; the object is the intent. The theft is not an act of defiance or anger. The differential diagnosis includes: stealing during a manic episode, stealing for actual gain, faking kleptomania (malingering) to avoid prosecution for stealing, conduct disorder in children and antisocial personality disorder in adults, both of which are associated with many other behavioral problems.

1. Fadem,B., Simring, S. High Yield Psychiatry. 2nd Edition. Lippincott, Williams & Wilkins, Philadelphia PA. 2003:101.

2. Kaplan, HI., Sadock BJ. A Comprehensive Textbook of Psychiatry. Williams & Wilkins, Baltimore MD. 1999:1701-1722.

93.   E   Intermittent explosive disorder

Intermittent explosive disorder is characterized by episodes in which the patient loses self-control and attacks another person without adequate cause. It was formerly called "episodic dyscontrol syndrome." The etiology is decreased serotonergic activity reflected in reduced levels of 5-hydroxyindoleacetic acid (5-HIAA), resulting in impulsivity. Treatment includes anticonvulsants (eg carbamazepine), and SSRIs. The differential diagnosis includes: alcohol or drug intoxication, loss of touch with reality (psychosis or dementia),

Medtext Medical World, Inc.

conduct disorder, antisocial personality disorder, and dissociate disorder (e.g., dissociative symptoms occur in "amok", a single episode of explosive behavior seen most commonly in Southeast Asia).

1. Fadem,B., Simring, S. High Yield Psychiatry. 2nd Edition. Lippincott, Williams & Wilkins, Philadelphia PA. 2003:103.

2. Kaplan, HI., Sadock BJ. A Comprehensive Textbook of Psychiatry. Williams & Wilkins, Baltimore MD. 1999:1701-1722.

94.   D   Trichotillomania

Trichotillomania is an impulse control disorder. Patients with trichotillomania have a need to pull out their hair. The result is obvious hair loss. Some also show trichophagia (hair eating), resulting in bezoars (hair balls), which can obstruct the bowel. The differential diagnosis includes alopecia caused by a medical condition and obsessive-compulsive disorder, which is not limited to one compulsion.

1. Kaplan, HI., Sadock BJ. A Comprehensive Textbook of Psychiatry. Williams & Wilkins, Baltimore MD. 1999:1701-1722.

95.   A   Pathological gambling

Pathological gambling is an impulse control disorder. Patients with pathological gambling have an overwhelming need to gamble that negatively affects family and work relationships. It is associated with loss of parent before or during adolescence, childhood attention-deficit/hyperactivity disorder, and major depressive disorder. The differential diagnosis includes a manic episode in which there is obvious elevation of mood. Pathological gambling is seen in up to 3% of adults, higher in late teens and early 20s.

1. Fadem,B., Simring, S. High Yield Psychiatry. 2nd Edition. Lippincott, Williams & Wilkins, Philadelphia PA. 2003:103.

2. Kaplan, HI., Sadock BJ. A Comprehensive Textbook of Psychiatry. Williams & Wilkins, Baltimore MD. 1999:1701-1722.

96.   C   Bereavement

After a major loss, a normal grief reaction can be expected to occur. Normal grief reaction (bereavement) is characterized by expected strong emotional response, usually sadness, after a loss (e.g., death of loved one, abortion, stillbirth, loss of a body part). Symptoms in normal grief include minor weight loss, mild sleep disturbance, mild guilt, illusions, and attempts to return to work and social activities, and expressions of sadness. After a major loss, normal grief or bereavement must be distinguished from abnormal grief or depression. Adjustment disorder occurs when a person who has experienced a stressful life event and show a maladaptive response (eg inhibited social interactions, problems at work) not seen in this case scenario.

1. Fadem,B., Simring, S. High Yield Psychiatry. 2nd Edition. Lippincott, Williams & Wilkins, Philadelphia PA. 2003:105.

2. Kaplan, HI., Sadock BJ. A Comprehensive Textbook of Psychiatry. Williams & Wilkins, Baltimore MD. 1999:1714-1721.

97.   A   Adjustment disorder

People who experience a stressful life event show either a normal response or a maladaptive disorder. In adjustment disorder, emotional symptoms begin within 3 months and end within 6 months of exposure to a psychological stressor; the intensity of the symptoms does not always correlate with the severity of the stressor. Impairment may be seen in occupational, academic, or social functioning. Adjustment disorder is common and is diagnosed in 2-8% of children, adolescents, and the elderly. It is present in 10-30% of mental health outpatients and is more common in disadvantaged populations.

1. Fadem,B., Simring, S. High Yield Psychiatry. 2nd Edition. Lippincott, Williams & Wilkins, Philadelphia PA. 2003:105.

2. Kaplan, HI., Sadock BJ. A Comprehensive Textbook of Psychiatry. Williams & Wilkins, Baltimore MD. 1999:1714-1722.

98.   A   Paranoid personality disorder

Personality disorders are pervasive, fixed, inappropriate patterns of relating to others that cause social and occupational impairment. The patients with paranoid personality disorder are characterized as distrustful, suspicious, litigious; attributes responsibility for own problems to others. Paranoid personality disorder is a Cluster A disorder where patients are characterized as peculiar, fear social relationships, genetic or familial association with psychotic illness. The other Cluster A disorders are schizoid personality disorder and schizotypal personality disorder. Psychodynamic mechanisms used by patients with paranoid personality disorder are denial (psychologically blocking out intolerable facts about reality) and projection (attributing one's unconscious, unacceptable impulses to others).

1. Fadem,B., Simring, S. High Yield Psychiatry. 2nd Edition. Lippincott, Williams & Wilkins, Philadelphia PA. 2003:108.

2. Kaplan, HI., Sadock BJ. A Comprehensive Textbook of Psychiatry. Williams & Wilkins, Baltimore MD. 1999:1723-1764.

99.   B   Schizoid personality disorder

Schizoid personality disorder is characterized by long-standing pattern of voluntary social withdrawal without psychosis. Schizoid personality disorder must be differentiated from delusional disorder, schizophrenia, Asperger disorder, and schizophrenia. Schizoid personality disorder is a Cluster A personality disorder. Cluster A also includes paranoid personality disorder and schizotypal personality disorder. In general, patients with personality disorders do not seek psychological help unless compelled by others, they do not have a frank psychosis, and the usually do not have disabling psychiatric symptoms.

1. Fadem,B., Simring, S. High Yield Psychiatry. 2nd Edition. Lippincott, Williams & Wilkins, Philadelphia PA. 2003:108.

2. Kaplan, HI., Sadock BJ. A Comprehensive Textbook of Psychiatry. Williams & Wilkins, Baltimore MD. 1999:1723-1764.

100.   **A**   **Dependent personality disorder**

Each personality disorder affects approximately 1% of the population, although many patients have features of more than one personality disorder. Dependent, histrionic, and schizotypal personality disorders are more common; schizoid personality disorder is less common. The dependent personality allows other people to make decisions and assume responsibility for them because of poor self-confidence. They may be abused by a domestic partner. Psychodynamic mechanisms used by patients with dependent personality disorder are regression (pushing unacceptable feelings into the unconscious) and avoidance.

1. Fadem,B., Simring, S. High Yield Psychiatry. 2nd Edition. Lippincott, Williams & Wilkins, Philadelphia PA. 2003:109.

2. Kaplan, HI., Sadock BJ. A Comprehensive Textbook of Psychiatry. Williams & Wilkins, Baltimore MD. 1999:1723-1764.

101.   **C**   **Histrionic personality disorder**

Patients with histrionic personality disorder are characterized as theatrical, extroverted, emotional, sexually provocative, "life of the party." They cannot maintain intimate relationships. When the disorder is present in men, "Don Juan" dress and behavior is commonly seen. Psychodynamic mechanisms exhibited in histrionic personality disorder include repression (pushing unacceptable feelings into the unconsciousness), regression (adopting childlike behavioral patterns), and somatization (physical symptoms without a sufficient organic cause). Individual and group psychotherapy and self-help groups may be useful.

1. Fadem,B., Simring, S. High Yield Psychiatry. 2nd Edition. Lippincott, Williams & Wilkins, Philadelphia PA. 2003:108.

2. Kaplan, HI., Sadock BJ. A Comprehensive Textbook of Psychiatry. Williams & Wilkins, Baltimore MD. 1999:1723-1764.

102.   C   Obsessive compulsive personality disorder

Personality disorders are chronic and life-long. Obsessive compulsive disorder is a Cluster C disorder. The other Cluster C disorders are avoidant, dependent, and passive-aggressive personality disorder (although passive-aggressive personality disorder is no longer an official DSM-IV-TR diagnosis). The obsessive compulsive personality is characterized as perfectionistic, orderly, stubborn, and indecisive with feelings of imperfection. Differential diagnosis includes obsessive-compulsive anxiety disorder. Psychodynamic mechanisms used by patients with obsessive compulsive personality disorder include isolation of affect (neither experiencing nor expressing emotions associated with stressful events), rationalization (giving seemingly reasonable explanations for unacceptable feelings), intellectualization (explaining away unwanted emotions), and undoing (attempting to reverse past actions by current actions).

1. Fadem,B., Simring, S. High Yield Psychiatry. 2nd Edition. Lippincott, Williams & Wilkins, Philadelphia PA. 2003:109.

2. Kaplan, HI., Sadock BJ. A Comprehensive Textbook of Psychiatry. Williams & Wilkins, Baltimore MD. 1999:1722-1764.

103.   A   Antisocial personality disorder

Antisocial personality is one who refuses to conform to social norms, shows no concern for others, and does not learn from experience. It is associated with conduct disorder in childhood and criminal behavior in adulthood. Antisocial personality disorder cannot be diagnosed until the patient is at least 18 years old. Before age 18, the diagnosis is conduct disorder. The psychodynamic mechanism exhibited by patients with antisocial personality disorder is inadequate superego functioning.

1. Fadem,B., Simring, S. High Yield Psychiatry. 2nd Edition. Lippincott, Williams & Wilkins, Philadelphia PA. 2003:109.

2. Kaplan, HI., Sadock BJ. A Comprehensive Textbook of Psychiatry. Williams & Wilkins, Baltimore MD. 1999:1722-1764.

104. **B** **Schizotypal personality disorder**

Patients with schizotypal personality are characterized by having a peculiar appearance, magical thinking, odd thought patterns and behavior without psychosis. Schizotypal personality disorder is a Cluster A disorder where patients are characterized as peculiar, fearful of social relationships, and have a genetic or familial association with psychotic illness. Schizotypal personality disorder is one of the more common personality disorders, along with histrionic and dependent personality disorders. Differential diagnosis includes delusional disorder, schizophrenia, and mood disorder with psychotic features. Not uncommonly patients also have major depressive disorder.

1. Fadem,B., Simring, S. High Yield Psychiatry. 2nd Edition. Lippincott, Williams & Wilkins, Philadelphia PA. 2003:108.

2. Kaplan, HI., Sadock BJ. A Comprehensive Textbook of Psychiatry. Williams & Wilkins, Baltimore MD. 1999:1722-1764.

105. **B** **Narcissistic personality disorder**

Narcissistic personality disorder is a Cluster B personality disorder. Patients with Cluster B personality disorders are characterized as emotional, inconsistent, or dramatic and have a genetic or familial association with mood disorders, substance abuse, and somatoform disorders. The other Cluster B disorders are histrionic, antisocial, and borderline personality disorders. Narcissistic personality is characterized as pompous, with a sense of special entitlement; lacks empathy for others. Psychodynamic mechanisms used by patients with narcissistic personality disorder are denial (psychologically blocking out intolerable facts about reality), displacement (transferring emotions from an unacceptable to a tolerable person or situation), and poor ego functioning.

1. Fadem,B., Simring, S. High Yield Psychiatry. 2nd Edition. Lippincott, Williams & Wilkins, Philadelphia PA. 2003:108.

2. Kaplan, HI., Sadock BJ. A Comprehensive Textbook of Psychiatry. Williams & Wilkins, Baltimore MD. 1999:1722-1764.

106.   C   Avoidant personality disorder

Avoidant personality disorder is a Cluster C personality disorder. Patients with Cluster C personality disorders are characterized as fearful, anxious, and have a genetic or familial association with anxiety disorders. The other Cluster C disorders are obsessive-compulsive, dependent and passive-aggressive personality disorders (although passive aggressive personality disorder is no longer considered an official DSM-IV-TR diagnosis). Avoidant personality is characterized as timid to rejection, and socially withdrawn with frequent feelings of inferiority. Psychodynamic mechanisms used by patients with avoidant personality disorder are displacement (transferring emotions from an unacceptable to a tolerable person or situation), regression (adopting childlike behavioral patterns), and avoidance.

1. Fadem,B., Simring, S. High Yield Psychiatry. 2nd Edition. Lippincott, Williams & Wilkins, Philadelphia PA. 2003:109.

2. Kaplan, HI., Sadock BJ. A Comprehensive Textbook of Psychiatry. Williams & Wilkins, Baltimore MD. 1999:1723-1764.

107.   B   Borderline personality disorder

Characteristics of borderline personality are erratic, unstable behavior and mood; boredom; feelings of aloneness; impulsiveness: suicide attempts; mini-psychotic episodes (e.g., brief periods of loss of contact with reality); self-mutilation (cutting or burning oneself without lethal intent). It is often co-morbid with mood disorders and eating disorders. Pharmacologic treatment is of limited use in personality disorders, except for borderline personality disorder, where antipsychotic or antidepressants may be necessary. Medication is used to treat associated target symptoms (e.g., depression, anxiety, mini-psychotic episodes). Medication must be prescribed cautiously (especially benzodiazepines) because many patients with personality disorders have a high potential for addiction.

1. Fadem,B., Simring, S. High Yield Psychiatry. 2nd Edition. Lippincott, Williams & Wilkins, Philadelphia PA. 2003:109.

2. Kaplan, HI., Sadock BJ. A Comprehensive Textbook of Psychiatry. Williams & Wilkins, Baltimore MD. 1999:1722-1764.

108.   **E**   **Passive aggressive personality disorder**

Passive-aggressive personality disorder is a Cluster C personality disorder where patients are characterized as fearful and anxious and have a genetic or familial association with anxiety disorders. The other Cluster C personality disorders are avoidant, obsessive-compulsive, and dependent personality disorders. Patients with passive-aggressive personality disorder are characterized as procrastinates, inefficient, outward compliance but inward defiance. The psychodynamic mechanism used by patients with passive aggressive personality disorder is reaction formation (denying unacceptable feelings and adopting opposite attitudes and behavior). Passive aggressive personality disorder was recently removed from the DSM-IV-TR diagnostic list.

1. Fadem,B., Simring, S. High Yield Psychiatry. 2nd Edition. Lippincott, Williams & Wilkins, Philadelphia PA. 2003:110.

2. Kaplan, HI., Sadock BJ. A Comprehensive Textbook of Psychiatry. Williams & Wilkins, Baltimore MD. 1999:1722-1764.

109.   **E**   **Androgens are associated with aggressiveness and agitation**

Androgens are non psychotropic agents that may cause psychiatric symptoms in some patients such as aggressiveness and agitation. Use of corticosteroids is associated with hypomania and euphoria. Abrupt withdrawal of corticosteroids is associated with depression, confusion, fatigue, headache, vomiting, pseudo-tumor cerebri like symptoms. Thyroid supplements are associated with anxiety and psychotic symptoms. Progestins are associated with depression and fatigue.

1. Fadem,B., Simring, S. High Yield Psychiatry. 2nd Edition. Lippincott, Williams & Wilkins, Philadelphia PA. 2003:119.

2. Kaplan, HI., Sadock BJ. A Comprehensive Textbook of Psychiatry. Williams & Wilkins, Baltimore MD. 1999:1577-1662.

Medtext Medical World, Inc.

110. **A** **Severe depression and confusion is associated with reserpine**

Psychiatric symptoms may be caused by non psychotropic agents, including antihypertensives. Nifedipine and verapamil have been associated with depression. Guanethidine, clonidine, methyldopa, and some diuretics are associated with mild depression, fatigue and sexual dysfunction. Beta-blockers (e.g. propranolol) have been associated with depression, fatigue, psychotic symptoms (less common). Reserpine is associated with severe depression and confusion.

1. Fadem,B., Simring, S. High Yield Psychiatry. 2nd Edition. Lippincott, Williams & Wilkins, Philadelphia PA. 2003:118.

2. Kaplan, HI., Sadock BJ. A Comprehensive Textbook of Psychiatry. Williams & Wilkins, Baltimore MD. 1999:1797-1803.

111. **C** **Chloramphenicol is associated with depression, confusion, and irritability**

Some drugs used to treat medical conditions such as antibiotics can precipitate psychiatric symptoms. Antituberculin agents (e.g., isoniazid) have been associated with psychotic symptoms (e.g., paranoia) and memory loss. Chloramphenicol and metronidazole have been associated with confusion, depression and irritability. Tetracycline has been associated with depression. Nitrofurantoin has been associated with confusion, headache, and sleepiness.

1. Fadem,B., Simring, S. High Yield Psychiatry. 2nd Edition. Lippincott, Williams & Wilkins, Philadelphia PA. 2003:118.

2. Kaplan, HI., Sadock BJ. A Comprehensive Textbook of Psychiatry. Williams & Wilkins, Baltimore MD. 1999:2235-2532.

112. **A** **Pentazocine has been associated with psychosis**

Medication-induced psychiatric symptoms occur with both psychotropic and non psychotropic medications. Pentazocine and propoxyphene have been associated with psychotic symptoms. Salicylates are associated with euphoria, depression, and confusion

Medtext Medical World, Inc.

(in very high doses). Indomethacin is associated with confusion, dizziness, psychotic symptoms, and depression (less common). Phenylbutazone is associated with anxiety.

1. Fadem,B., Simring, S. High Yield Psychiatry. 2nd Edition. Lippincott, Williams & Wilkins, Philadelphia PA. 2003:119.

2. Kaplan, HI., Sadock BJ. A Comprehensive Textbook of Psychiatry. Williams & Wilkins, Baltimore MD. 1999:2232-2532.

113.   **A**   **Patients on renal dialysis are at increased risk for psychological problems, in part because they must depend on other people and on machines**

Consult-liaison psychiatrists treat psychiatric problems in medical patients. Consult-liaison psychiatrists recommend specific psychotropic medications and provide psychosocial interventions. Hospitalized patients who are at the greatest risk for psychological problems include patients with acquired immune deficiency syndrome (AIDS), patients who are undergoing surgery, patients being treated in the ICU or CCU, and patients on renal dialysis. The most common psychological problems for renal dialysis patients are depression, suicide and sexual dysfunction. Both psychological and medical risk can be reduced through the use of in-home dialysis units, which cause less disruption of the patient's life.

1. Fadem,B., Simring, S. High Yield Psychiatry. 2nd Edition. Lippincott, Williams & Wilkins, Philadelphia PA. 2003:120.

2. Kaplan, HI., Sadock BJ. A Comprehensive Textbook of Psychiatry. Williams & Wilkins, Baltimore MD. 1999:1765-1887.

114.   **E**   **All of the above**

        The illness is potentially fatal
        Guilt for past high-risk behaviors
        Guilt for exposure of others to the virus
        Forced to 'come out" to others if homosexual

AIDS is potentially fatal. Patient may experience guilt because they engaged in behavior that led to the illness (e.g., sex with multiple partners, intravenous drug abuse) and may have given the virus to others. They must deal with others' fears of contagion.

Medtext Medical World, Inc.

Homosexual patients may be forced to "come out" (reveal their sexual orientation) to others. Psychological counseling can reduce psychological and medical risk.

1. Fadem,B., Simring, S. High Yield Psychiatry. 2nd Edition. Lippincott, Williams & Wilkins, Philadelphia PA. 2003:120.

2. Kaplan, HI., Sadock BJ. A Comprehensive Textbook of Psychiatry. Williams & Wilkins, Baltimore MD. 1999:1765-1887.

115.   A   Phenelzine

A patient on an MAO inhibitor who eats in an unfamiliar place (e.g., restaurant) may unwittingly ingest tyramine containing foods. MAO inhibitors irreversibly limit the activity of monoamine oxidase, increase the availability of norepinephrine and serotonin in the synapse, and improve mood. MAO metabolizes tyramine, a pressor, in the gastrointestinal tract. If MAO is inhibited, foods that are rich in tyramine (e.g., aged cheese, chicken or beef liver, smoked or pickled meats or fish, broad beans, beer, red wine) can increase the level of tyramine and cause a hypertensive crisis. Sympathomimetic drugs (e.g., ephedrine, methylphenidate, phenylephrine, and pseudoephedrine) can also increase the level of tyramine and cause a hypertensive crisis, which can lead to stroke and death.

1. Fadem,B., Simring, S. High Yield Psychiatry. 2nd Edition. Lippincott, Williams & Wilkins, Philadelphia PA. 2003:127.

2. Kaplan, HI., Sadock BJ. A Comprehensive Textbook of Psychiatry. Williams & Wilkins, Baltimore MD. 1999:2397.

116.   E   All of the above

Aged cheese
Chicken or beef liver
Smoked or pickled meat or fish
Beer or red wine

MAO inhibitors are used primarily to improve mood. They may also be used for atypical depression, panic disorder, eating disorders, pain disorders, and social phobia. If MAO is inhibited, foods that are rich in tyramine (e.g., aged cheese, chicken or beef liver, smoked or pickled meats or fish, broad beans, beer or red wine) can increase the level of tyramine resulting in hyperadrenergic crisis. MAO inhibitors and SSRIs used together can cause another potentially life-threatening drug-drug interaction, the serotonin syndrome. Serotonin syndrome is marked by autonomic instability, hyperthermia, convulsions, coma, and death.

C A H C

1. Fadem,B., Simring, S. High Yield Psychiatry. 2nd Edition. Lippincott, Williams & Wilkins, Philadelphia PA. 2003:127.

2. Kaplan, HI., Sadock BJ. A Comprehensive Textbook of Psychiatry. Williams & Wilkins, Baltimore MD. 1999:2397.

117.　　　D　　Ebstein's anomaly

Lithium is the primary treatment to abort the manic phase of bipolar disorder. Lithium is also a mood stabilizer that is used to prevent both the manic and the depressive phases of bipolar disorder. Lithium is also used to augment the effectiveness of antidepressant agents in depressive illness. Adverse effects associated with lithium include: first trimester congenital abnormalities (especially Ebstein's anomaly, a cardiac malformation), tremor, renal dysfunction, cardiac conduction problems, hypothyroidism, acne, gastric distress, mild cognitive impairment. Lithium takes 1 to 2 weeks to work.

1. Fadem,B., Simring, S. High Yield Psychiatry. 2nd Edition. Lippincott, Williams & Wilkins, Philadelphia PA. 2003:128.

2. Kaplan, HI., Sadock BJ. A Comprehensive Textbook of Psychiatry. Williams & Wilkins, Baltimore MD. 1999:2377-2389.

118.　　　A　　Congenital neural tube defects

Valproic acid is used, along with divalproex and the newer anticonvulsant agents, to treat bipolar disorder. These agents are used particularly to treat the mixed episode (e.g. mania and depression occurring in the same episode) and rapid cycling (at least four episodes of mania and depression yearly) types. Adverse effects associated with valproic acid include: gastrointestinal symptoms, liver problems, congenital neural tube defects, alopecia, weight gain. Psychomotor slowing, sedation, renal dysfunction, and thyroid dysfunction are not

Medtext Medical World, Inc.

associated with use of valproic acid. Valproic acid is an anticonvulsant and is also used to treat migraine headaches, bipolar symptoms resulting from cognitive disorders, mixed episode and rapid cycling bipolar disorder, impulse control disorders, and withdrawal from sedatives.

1. Fadem,B., Simring, S. High Yield Psychiatry. 2nd Edition. Lippincott, Williams & Wilkins, Philadelphia PA. 2003:128.

2. Kaplan, HI., Sadock BJ. A Comprehensive Textbook of Psychiatry. Williams & Wilkins, Baltimore MD. 1999:2289-2298.

119.   A   Aplastic anemia

Carbamazepine is a mood stabilizing agent. It is an anticonvulsant and may also be used to treat trigeminal neuralgia, impulse control disorders, and withdrawal from sedatives. Adverse effects associated with carbamazepine include aplastic anemia and agranulocytosis, which require monitoring. Additional adverse effects include sedation, dizziness, ataxia, and congenital anomalies. Neural tube defects, alopecia, hypothyroidism, and renal dysfunction are not associated with use of carbamazepine.

1. Fadem,B., Simring, S. High Yield Psychiatry. 2nd Edition. Lippincott, Williams & Wilkins, Philadelphia PA. 2003:128.

2. Kaplan, HI., Sadock BJ. A Comprehensive Textbook of Psychiatry. Williams & Wilkins, Baltimore MD. 1999:2282-2288.

120.   A   Psychomotor slowing

The newer anticonvulsants may have mood-stabilizing effects. These include topiramate (Topamax), lamotrigine (Lamictal), gabapentin (Neurontin), and tiagabine (Gabitril). The newer anticonvulsants, valproic acid, and divalproex are used to treat bipolar disorder, particularly the mixed episode and rapid cycling. Topiramate is associated with psychomotor slowing and fatigue. Topiramate is not associated with dizziness, ataxia, blood dyscrasia, or autoinduction.

1. Fadem,B., Simring, S. High Yield Psychiatry. 2nd Edition. Lippincott, Williams & Wilkins, Philadelphia PA. 2003:128.

2. Kaplan, HI., Sadock BJ. A Comprehensive Textbook of Psychiatry. (pp. 2299-2303) Williams & Wilkins, Baltimore MD. 1999:2299-2303.

121.   A   Dizziness, ataxia, visual disturbance

Oxcarbazepine (Trileptal) is a mood stabilizing agent. It is also an anticonvulsant and has been used to treat trigeminal neuralgia. Adverse effects associated with oxcarbazepine include: dizziness, ataxia, and visual disturbances. Unlike with use of carbamazepine, with oxcarbazepine there is no blood dyscrasia or autoinduction. Oxcarbazepine also not associated with cardiac conduction disturbance and mild renal impairments.

1. Fadem,B., Simring, S. High Yield Psychiatry. 2nd Edition. Lippincott, Williams & Wilkins, Philadelphia PA. 2003:128.

2. Kaplan, HI., Sadock BJ. A Comprehensive Textbook of Psychiatry. (pp. 2299-2302) Williams & Wilkins, Baltimore MD. 1999:2299-2302.

122.   A   Amoxapine

Amoxapine has both antidepressant and antipsychotic activity. Its adverse effects include: antidopaminergic effects like Parkinsonian symptoms, galactorrhea, and sexual dysfunction. It is considered the most dangerous antidepressant in overdose. Tranylcypromine is a monoamine oxidase inhibitor (MAOI) and its adverse effects are hyperadrenergic crisis, orthostatic hypotension, sexual dysfunction, and insomnia. Adverse effects of bupropion include insomnia, seizures, sweating, decreased appetite. Mirtazapine causes sedation. Venlafaxine has serotonergic and noradrenergic effects and increases diastolic blood pressure at high doses.

1. Fadem,B., Simring, S. High Yield Psychiatry. 2nd Edition. Lippincott, Williams & Wilkins, Philadelphia PA. 2003:128.

2. Kaplan, HI., Sadock BJ. A Comprehensive Textbook of Psychiatry. Williams & Wilkins, Baltimore MD. 1999:2356.

123.   B   Seizures

Bupropion is an antidepressant. Bupropion is associated with insomnia, seizures, sweating, and decreased appetite. It has fewer adverse sexual effects that other antidepressants. It is used to treat refractory depression (inadequate clinical response to other antidepressants), seasonal affective disorder (SAD), adult attention deficit hyperactivity disorder, and SSRI-induced sexual dysfunction. It has recently been used for smoking cessation.

1. Fadem,B., Simring, S. High Yield Psychiatry. 2nd Edition. Lippincott, Williams & Wilkins, Philadelphia PA. 2003:126.

2. Kaplan, HI., Sadock BJ. A Comprehensive Textbook of Psychiatry. Williams & Wilkins, Baltimore MD. 1999:2324-2328.

124. **A** **Increased diastolic blood pressure**

Venlafaxine is an antidepressant. Venlafaxine is associated with serotonergic and noradrenergic activity. It has low cytochrome P450 activity, increases diastolic blood pressure in high doses, has the highest remission rate, and has the fewest sexual side effects. It is indicated for refractory depression, having the fastest action working within 10 days. Amoxapine causes Parkinsonian effects. Bupropion decreases appetite. Monoamine oxidase inhibitors (phenelzine and tranylcypromine) cause orthostatic hypotension.

1. Fadem,B., Simring, S. High Yield Psychiatry. 2nd Edition. Lippincott, Williams & Wilkins, Philadelphia PA. 2003:126.

2. Kaplan, HI., Sadock BJ. A Comprehensive Textbook of Psychiatry. Williams & Wilkins, Baltimore MD. 1999:2427.

125. **E** **Impotence**

SSRIs selectively block the reuptake of serotonin, but have limited effects on the norepinephrine, dopamine, histamine and acetylcholine systems. Because of their selectivity, SSRIs cause fewer side effects and are safer in overdose than heterocyclics or MAO inhibitors. SSRIs have become the first-line treatment for most patients with depressive illness. Special clinical uses in addition to depression for SSRIs include: OCD, premature ejaculation, panic disorder, premenstrual dysphoric disorder, paraphilias, hypochondriasis, social phobia, chronic pain, PTSD, migraine headaches, and bulimia. Adverse effects of SSRIs include gastrointestinal disturbances, sexual dysfunction, agitation and insomnia.

1. Fadem,B., Simring, S. High Yield Psychiatry. 2nd Edition. Lippincott, Williams & Wilkins, Philadelphia PA. 2003:125.

2. Kaplan, HI., Sadock BJ. A Comprehensive Textbook of Psychiatry. Williams & Wilkins, Baltimore MD. 1999:2432.

126.   **E**   **Fluoxetine is associated with sexual dysfunction**

Fluoxetine may cause agitation and insomnia initially and is well associated with sexual dysfunction. Paroxetine and escitalopram are the most serotonin specific of the SSRIs. Paroxetine is associated with sexual dysfunction and escitalopram is reported to have less side-effect than citalopram. Fluvoxamine is currently only has FDA indication for OCD. Sertraline is the most likely SSRI to cause gastrointestinal side effects and is well associated with sexual dysfunction.

1. Fadem,B., Simring, S. High Yield Psychiatry. 2nd Edition. Lippincott, Williams & Wilkins, Philadelphia PA. 2003:125.

2. Kaplan, HI., Sadock BJ. A Comprehensive Textbook of Psychiatry. Williams & Wilkins, Baltimore MD. 1999:2432.

127.   **C**   **Maprotiline has low cardiotoxicity**

Heterocyclic antidepressants include amitriptyline, clomipramine, desipramine, doxepin, imipramine, maprotiline, and nortriptyline. Maprotiline has low cardiotoxicity and may cause seizures. Nortriptyline is the least likely to cause orthostatic hypotension. Amitriptyline is highly sedating and anticholinergic. Clomipramine is the most serotonin specific of the heterocyclics. Imipramine is likely to cause orthostatic hypotension. Desipramine is the least sedating and least anticholinergic.

1. Fadem,B., Simring, S. High Yield Psychiatry. 2nd Edition. Lippincott, Williams & Wilkins, Philadelphia PA. 2003:125.

2. Kaplan, HI., Sadock BJ. A Comprehensive Textbook of Psychiatry. Williams & Wilkins, Baltimore MD. 1999:2491.

Medtext Medical World, Inc.

128. **E** **Olanzapine for negative symptoms**

Perphenazine has been used for nausea and emesis but not for body dysmorphic disorder. Pimozide has been used for Tourette disorder and body dysmorphic disorder. Trifluoperazine has been used for nonpsychotic anxiety (may be used for as long as 12 weeks), but is not available in long-acting (decanoate) form. Fluphenazine, haloperidol and risperidone are available in long-acting (decanoate) formulations. Chlorpromazine has been used for nausea, emesis and hiccups.

1. Fadem,B., Simring, S. High Yield Psychiatry. 2nd Edition. Lippincott, Williams & Wilkins, Philadelphia PA. 2003:124.

2. Kaplan, HI., Sadock BJ. A Comprehensive Textbook of Psychiatry. Williams & Wilkins, Baltimore MD. 1999:2455.

129. **C** **Sublimation**

Altruism, humor, sublimation and suppression are "mature" defense mechanisms because, when used to moderation, they directly help the patient or others. Denial, projection, and splitting are most often pathological defense mechanisms. Denial is not accepting aspects of reality that the individual finds unbearable. Projection is attributing one's unacceptable feelings to others. Splitting is categorizing people (or even the same person at different time) as either "perfect" or "awful"; an intolerance of ambiguity. Lying is not considered to be a defense mechanism.

1. Fadem,B., Simring, S. High Yield Psychiatry. 2nd Edition. Lippincott, Williams & Wilkins, Philadelphia PA. 2003:131.

2. Kaplan, HI., Sadock BJ. A Comprehensive Textbook of Psychiatry. Williams & Wilkins, Baltimore MD. 1999:563-606.

130. **A** **Isolation of affect**

Defense mechanisms are unconscious mental techniques used by the mind to keep conflicts out of awareness, reduce anxiety, and maintain a person's self-esteem and sense of safety and equilibrium. The mechanisms are enacted by the "ego" component of the mind. Isolation of affect is characterized by failure to experience the feelings associated with a stressful life event, although the person logically understands the significance of the event. Rationalization is distorting one's perception of an event so that its negative outcome seems reasonable. Dissociation is mentally separating part of one's consciousness or mentally distancing oneself from others. Displacement is moving emotions from a personally unacceptable situation to one that is personally tolerable.

1. Fadem,B., Simring, S. High Yield Psychiatry. 2nd Edition. Lippincott, Williams & Wilkins, Philadelphia PA. 2003:133.

2. Kaplan, HI., Sadock BJ. A Comprehensive Textbook of Psychiatry. Williams & Wilkins, Baltimore MD. 1999:563-606.

131. B Rationalization

Rationalization is characterized by distorting one's perception of an event so that its negative outcome seems reasonable. Isolation of affect is failing to experience the feelings associated with a stressful life event, although the person logically understands the significance of the event. Help-rejecting complaining is dealing with emotional conflict by complaining or molding repetitious requests for help that disguise covert feelings of hostility or reproach towards others, which are then expressed by rejecting the suggestions, advice, or help that others offer. Affiliation is dealing with emotional conflict or internal or external stressors by turning to others for help or support. Humor is expressing feelings without causing discomfort.

1. Fadem,B., Simring, S. High Yield Psychiatry. 2nd Edition. Lippincott, Williams & Wilkins, Philadelphia PA. 2003:133.

2. Kaplan, HI., Sadock BJ. A Comprehensive Textbook of Psychiatry. Williams & Wilkins, Baltimore MD. 1999:563-606.

132. C Projection

Projection is characterized as attributing one's unacceptable feelings to others; associated with paranoid symptoms and ordinary jealousy. Defensive jealousy is not a specific defense mechanism. Intellectualization is using the mind's higher functions to avoid experiencing emotion and is associated with obsessive-compulsive personality disorder. Projection is attributing one's unacceptable feeling to others and is associated with paranoid symptoms and ordinary prejudice. Anticipation is dealing with emotional conflict by experiencing emotional reactions in advance of, or anticipating consequences of, possible future events and considering realistic, alternative responses or solutions. Acting out is avoiding unacceptable emotions by behaving in an attention-getting, often socially inappropriate manner.

1. Fadem,B., Simring, S. High Yield Psychiatry. 2nd Edition. Lippincott, Williams & Wilkins, Philadelphia PA. 2003:133.

2. Kaplan, HI., Sadock BJ. A Comprehensive Textbook of Psychiatry. Williams & Wilkins, Baltimore MD. 1999:563-606.

133.   E   Intellectualization

Intellectualization is marked by using the mind's higher functions to avoid experiencing emotion and is associated with obsessive-compulsive personality disorder. Sublimation is expressing an unacceptable impulse in a socially useful way. Identification (with the aggressor) is patterning one's behavior after that of someone more powerful; it may be positive or negative. Tolerance is not considered to be a defense mechanism. Undoing is believing that one can magically reverse events caused by "wrong" behavior by adopting "right" behavior.

1. Fadem,B., Simring, S. High Yield Psychiatry. 2nd Edition. Lippincott, Williams & Wilkins, Philadelphia PA. 2003:133.

2. Kaplan, HI., Sadock BJ. A Comprehensive Textbook of Psychiatry. Williams & Wilkins, Baltimore MD. 1999:563-606.

134.   C   Identification

Identification (with the aggressor) is characterized by patterning one's behavior after that of someone more powerful (may be positive or negative). Reaction formation is adopting opposite attitudes to avoid unacceptable emotions; unlike hypocrisy, this is an unconscious behavior. Sublimation is expressing an unacceptable impulse in a socially useful way. Dissociation is mentally separating part of one's consciousness or mentally distancing oneself from others. Idealization is when the individual deals with emotional conflict by attributing exaggerated positive qualities to others.

1. Fadem,B., Simring, S. High Yield Psychiatry. 2nd Edition. Lippincott, Williams & Wilkins, Philadelphia PA. 2003:133.

2. Kaplan, HI., Sadock BJ. A Comprehensive Textbook of Psychiatry. Williams & Wilkins, Baltimore MD. 1999:563-606.

135.   A   Humor

Humor as a defense mechanism is characterized by expressing feelings without causing discomfort. Altruism is assisting others in order to avoid negative personal feeling. Splitting is categorizing people (or even the same person at different times) as either "perfect" or "awful"; an intolerance of ambiguity. Reaction negotiation is not considered to be a defense mechanism. Undoing is believing that one can magically reverse events caused by "wrong" behavior by adopting "right" behavior.

1. Fadem,B., Simring, S. High Yield Psychiatry. 2nd Edition. Lippincott, Williams & Wilkins, Philadelphia PA. 2003:133.

2. Kaplan, HI., Sadock BJ. A Comprehensive Textbook of Psychiatry. Williams & Wilkins, Baltimore MD. 1999:563-606.

136. **B** **Displacement**

Displacement is characterized by moving emotions from a personally unacceptable situation to one that is personally tolerable. Suppression is deliberately pushing unacceptable emotions out of conscious awareness. Regression is reverting to behavior pattern typical of a younger person and is seen in patients with dependent personality disorder. Devaluation is the individual dealing with emotional conflict or internal or external stressors by attributing exaggerated negative qualities to self or others. Self-assertion is dealing with emotional conflict by expressing his or her own thoughts, feeling, motivation and behavior, and responding appropriately.

1. Fadem,B., Simring, S. High Yield Psychiatry. 2nd Edition. Lippincott, Williams & Wilkins, Philadelphia PA. 2003:133.

2. Kaplan, HI., Sadock BJ. A Comprehensive Textbook of Psychiatry. Williams & Wilkins, Baltimore MD. 1999:563-606.

137. **A** **Denial**

Denial as a defense mechanism is marked by not accepting aspects of reality that the individual finds unbearable. Autistic fantasy is dealing with emotional conflict by excessive daydreaming as a substitute for human relationships, more effective action, or problem solving. Self-observation is dealing with emotional conflict by reflecting on his or her own thoughts, feeling, motivation, and behavior, and responding accordingly. Self accusation and self initiation are not recognized defense mechanisms.

1. Fadem,B., Simring, S. High Yield Psychiatry. 2nd Edition. Lippincott, Williams & Wilkins, Philadelphia PA. 2003:133.

2. Kaplan, HI., Sadock BJ. A Comprehensive Textbook of Psychiatry. Williams & Wilkins, Baltimore MD. 1999:563-606.

Medtext Medical World, Inc.

138.   **E**   **Acting out**

Acting out as a defense mechanism is characterized by avoiding unacceptable emotions by behaving in an attention-getting, often socially inappropriate manner. Self-observation is dealing with emotional conflict by reflecting on his or her own thoughts, feeling, motivation, and behavior, and responding appropriately. Omnipotence is the dealing with emotional conflict by feeling or acting as if he or she possesses special powers or abilities and is superior to others. Passive aggression is dealing with emotional conflict by indirectly and unassertively expressing aggression toward others. Misidentification of the aggression is not a recognized defense mechanism.

1. Fadem,B., Simring, S. High Yield Psychiatry. 2nd Edition. Lippincott, Williams & Wilkins, Philadelphia PA. 2003:133.

2. Kaplan, HI., Sadock BJ. A Comprehensive Textbook of Psychiatry. Williams & Wilkins, Baltimore MD. 1999:563-606.

139.   **E**   **Altruism**

Altruism as a defense mechanism is marked by assisting others in order to avoid negative personal feelings. Self-assertion is dealing with emotional conflict by expressing his or her feelings and thoughts directly in a way that is not coercive or manipulative. Help-rejecting complaining is dealing with emotional conflict by complaining or molding repetitious requests for help that disguise covert feelings of hostility or reproach toward others, which are then expressed by rejecting the suggestions, advice, or help that others offer. Projective identification is dealing with emotional conflict by falsely attributing to another his or her own unacceptable feelings, impulses, or thoughts; unlike simple projection, the individual does not fully disavow what is projected and instead remains aware of his or her own affects or impulses by misattributes them as justifiable reactions to the other person. Suppression is dealing with emotional conflict by intentionally avoiding thinking about disturbing problems, wishes, feelings, or experiences.

1. Fadem,B., Simring, S. High Yield Psychiatry. 2nd Edition. Lippincott, Williams & Wilkins, Philadelphia PA. 2003:133.

2. Kaplan, HI., Sadock BJ. A Comprehensive Textbook of Psychiatry. Williams & Wilkins, Baltimore MD. 1999:563-606.

140. **C** **Reaction formation**

Reaction formation as a defense mechanism is characterized by adopting opposite attitudes to avoid unacceptable emotions; unlike hypocrisy, this is an unconscious process. Autistic fantasy is dealing with emotional conflict by excessive daydreaming as a substitute for human relationships, more effective action, or problem solving. Antisocial behavior is not considered to be a defense mechanism. Anticipation is dealing with emotional conflict by experiencing emotional reactions in advance of, or anticipating consequences of, possible future events and considering realistic, alternative responses or solutions. Devaluation is dealing with emotional conflict by attributing exaggerated negative qualities to self or others.

1. Fadem,B., Simring, S. High Yield Psychiatry. 2nd Edition. Lippincott, Williams & Wilkins, Philadelphia PA. 2003:134.

2. Kaplan, HI., Sadock BJ. A Comprehensive Textbook of Psychiatry. Williams & Wilkins, Baltimore MD. 1999:563-606.

141. **E** **Regression**

Regression is marked by reverting to behavior patterns typical of a younger person; seen in patients with dependent personality disorder. Possessiveness is not considered to be a defense mechanism. Idealization is dealing with emotional conflict by attributing exaggerated positive qualities to others. Affiliation is dealing with emotional conflict by turning to others for help or support. Passive aggression is dealing with emotional conflicts by indirectly and unassertively expressing aggression toward others.

1. Fadem,B., Simring, S. High Yield Psychiatry. 2nd Edition. Lippincott, Williams & Wilkins, Philadelphia PA. 2003:134.

2. Kaplan, HI., Sadock BJ. A Comprehensive Textbook of Psychiatry. Williams & Wilkins, Baltimore MD. 1999:563-606.

142.   **B**   **Counter-transference**

The central strategy of psychoanalysis is to slowly uncover experiences that are repressed in the unconscious mind. These experiences are then reintegrated into the patient's personality. Counter-transference is the psychological phenomenon marked by unconscious re-experiencing of feeling about parents or other important figures in the therapist's life in her current relationship with the patient. Transference is the unconscious re-experiencing of feelings about parents or important figures in the patient's life in his current relationship with the therapist. Transference and counter transference are phenomena that occur during psychoanalysis as well as in ordinary physician-patient relationships.

1. Fadem,B., Simring, S. High Yield Psychiatry. 2nd Edition. Lippincott, Williams & Wilkins, Philadelphia PA. 2003:134.

2. Kaplan, HI., Sadock BJ. A Comprehensive Textbook of Psychiatry. Williams & Wilkins, Baltimore MD. 1999:563-606.

143.   **A**   **Transference**

Psychoanalysis uses a number of techniques to recover repressed memories. Free-association is when a patient lies on a couch facing away from the therapist and says whatever comes to mind. Layer by layer, unconscious memories are revealed and the therapist interprets the information. Analysis of resistance (the blocking of unconscious thoughts from consciousness because the patient finds them unacceptable), interpretation of dreams (the representation of conflict between fears and wishes), and analysis of transference (the patient's reaction to the therapist) are additional techniques. Transference is the psychological phenomenon marked by unconscious re-experiencing of feelings about parents or important figures in the patient's life in his current relationship with the therapist.

1. Fadem,B., Simring, S. High Yield Psychiatry. 2nd Edition. Lippincott, Williams & Wilkins, Philadelphia PA. 2003:134.

2. Kaplan, HI., Sadock BJ. A Comprehensive Textbook of Psychiatry. Williams & Wilkins, Baltimore MD. 1999:563-606.

144.   D   Splitting

Personality disorders are pervasive, fixed inappropriate patterns of relating to others that cause social and occupational impairment. Patients with personality disorders typically have limited insight, do not seek psychological help, do not have frank psychosis, and do not have disabling psychiatric symptoms. Splitting is a defense mechanism marked by categorizing people (or even the same person at different times) as either "perfect" or "awful"; intolerance of ambiguity. Splitting is seen in patients with borderline personality disorder. Other psychodynamic mechanisms used by patients with borderline personality disorder are denial, displacement, and poor ego functioning.

1. Fadem,B., Simring, S. High Yield Psychiatry. 2nd Edition. Lippincott, Williams & Wilkins, Philadelphia PA. 2003:134.

2. Kaplan, HI., Sadock BJ. A Comprehensive Textbook of Psychiatry. Williams & Wilkins, Baltimore MD. 1999:563-606.

145.   A   Sublimation

Psychoanalysis and related therapies are based on Freud's ideal that behavior is determined by forces derived from unconscious mental processes. Although defense mechanisms protect the patient, if any one is used exclusively or excessively, neurotic symptoms will result. Sublimation is one of the "mature" defense mechanisms along with altruism, humor, and suppression. When used in moderation, the "mature" defense mechanisms directly help the patient or others. Sublimation is marked by the expression of unacceptable impulses in a socially useful way.

1. Fadem,B., Simring, S. High Yield Psychiatry. 2nd Edition. Lippincott, Williams & Wilkins, Philadelphia PA. 2003:134.

2. Kaplan, HI., Sadock BJ. A Comprehensive Textbook of Psychiatry. Williams & Wilkins, Baltimore MD. 1999:563-606.

146. **C** **Undoing**

Defense mechanisms are enacted by the "ego" component of the mind. Freud's early (topographic) and later (structural) theories of the mind were developed to explain his ideals. The ego is part of Freud's structural theory, which includes id, ego, and superego as the functional components of the mind. The ego begins to develop immediately after birth and controls the expression of instinctual drives, primarily by the use of defense mechanisms to adapt to the requirement of the external work. The ego also: maintains a relationship with the external world, evaluates what is valid, adapts to that reality, and maintains satisfying interpersonal or object relations. Undoing is a defense mechanism marked by the belief that one can magically reverse events caused by "wrong" behavior by adopting "right" behavior.

1. Fadem,B., Simring, S. High Yield Psychiatry. 2nd Edition. Lippincott, Williams & Wilkins, Philadelphia PA. 2003:134.

2. Kaplan, HI., Sadock BJ. A Comprehensive Textbook of Psychiatry. Williams & Wilkins, Baltimore MD. 1999:563-606.

147. **C** **Repression**

The fundamental defense mechanism is repression; all other defense mechanisms are based on repression. In repression, the patient deals with emotional conflict by expelling disturbing wishes, thoughts, or experiences from conscious awareness. The feeling component may remain conscious, detached from its associated ideas. In Freud's topographic (early) theory of the mind, the components of the mind include the unconscious, the preconscious, and the conscious. The unconscious contains repressed thoughts and feelings, using primary process thinking (e.g., has no logic or concept of time, and involves primitive drives, wish fulfillment, and pleasure seeking). Primary process thinking is also common in young children and psychotic adults.

1. Fadem,B., Simring, S. High Yield Psychiatry. 2nd Edition. Lippincott, Williams & Wilkins, Philadelphia PA. 2003:134.

2. Kaplan, HI., Sadock BJ. A Comprehensive Textbook of Psychiatry. Williams & Wilkins, Baltimore MD. 1999:563-606.

 Medtext Medical World, Inc.

148. **A** **Id**

Freud's structural (later) theories of the mind include the id, ego, and superego as the primary components of the mind. The id is present at birth and is controlled by primary process thinking. It contains instinctual sexual and aggressive drives. The id acts in concert with the pleasure principle and is not influenced by external reality. It operates almost completely on an unconscious level.

2. Kaplan, HI., Sadock BJ. A Comprehensive Textbook of Psychiatry. Williams & Wilkins, Baltimore MD. 1999:563-606.

149. **C** **Superego**

Psychoanalysis and related therapies are based on Freud's idea that behavior is determined by forces derived from unconscious mental processes. Freud's structural (later) theories of the mind include the id, ego, and superego as the primary components of the mind. The superego is developed by approximately 6 years of age. It is associated with conscience and morality. The superego operates on unconscious, preconscious, and conscious levels.

1. Fadem,B., Simring, S. High Yield Psychiatry. 2nd Edition. Lippincott, Williams & Wilkins, Philadelphia PA. 2003:132.

2. Kaplan, HI., Sadock BJ. A Comprehensive Textbook of Psychiatry. Williams & Wilkins, Baltimore MD. 1999:563-606.

150. **C** **Nicotine replacement therapy does not cause acute vascular injury**

The case describes a low degree of nicotine dependence. Nicotine replacement therapy in contrast to smoking does not cause acute vascular injury. The use of Bupropion and nicotine is relatively safe but contraindicated in patients with seizures and in eating disorders. Nicotine replacement therapy prevents withdrawal and also maintains nicotine relaxing effects. Nicotine replacement therapies have been estimated to double smoking cessation rates. Replacement therapies use a short period of maintenance (6 to 12 weeks) often followed by a gradual reduction period (6 to 12 weeks).

Medtext Medical World, Inc.

The stimulating effects of nicotine produce improved attention, learning, reaction time and problem solving capability. Short–term nicotine exposure increases cerebral blood flow (CBF) without affecting cerebral oxygen metabolism. Studies have shown that combining nicotine replacement and behavior therapy increase the rate of smoking cessation than either therapy alone.

1. Gabbard GO. Treatments of Psychiatric Disorders, 3rd edition. American Psychiatric Publishing Inc. Washington DC. 2001:766-9

2. Sadock BJ, Sadock VA. Kaplan & Sadock's Synopsis of Psychiatry, 9th edition. Lippincott, Williams & Wilkins, Philadelphia, PA. 2003:444-448.

151.   D   It can precede substance abuse 85% of the time

Alcohol use causes a transient relaxing effect and a temporary relief from shyness. The anxiety can either be discrete (specific) limited to a certain situation or generalized (like public speaking, performing, eating, etc.) Patients usually fear being labeled as crazy or psycho due to their degree of severe anxiety in social situations. Social phobia is common in patients with avoidant personality disorder. Patients with social phobia may have a history of other anxiety disorders, mood disorders, substance-related disorders and bulimia nervosa. The peak age of social phobia onset is during the teen years; however onset is common as young as 5 years of age and as old as 31 years.

1. Hales RE, Yudofsky SC. Textbook of Clinical Psychiatry, 4th edition. American Psychiatric Publishing Inc. Washington DC. 2003:572-9.

152.   A   The combination with alcohol has teratogenic effect

The combination with alcohol can lead to hypotension, which may decrease placental perfusion. Disulfiram has dopaminergic action and can cause psychosis.

1. Sadock BJ, Sadock V. Kaplan & Sadock's Comprehensive Textbook of Psychiatry, 7th edition. Lippincott, Williams & Wilkins. New York NY. 2000:970,2243,2529.

2.Krulewitch CJ. An unexpected adverse drug effect. *Journal of Midwifery Women Health* 2003;48(1):67-8

153.   **A**   **Rivastigmine**

Cholinesterase inhibitors are usually referred to as anti-dementia medications. Rivastigmine is available in capsule and oral solution forms. Galantamine is available in capsule and oral solution. Donepezil is a tablet and tacrine is a capsule. Risperidone is an atypical antipsychotic available in tablets, in orally disintegrated tablets, and in a solution form, and is sometime used in the management of behavioral and psychosis in patients with dementia. It is not considered an anti-dementia medication. Risperidone has been most recently approved in a long acting intramuscular formula for the treatment of non compliance in patients with schizophrenia.

1. Physicians' Desk Reference, 58th edition. Thomson PDR. Montvale NJ. 2004:1759,1764,2255.

2. Doody RS. Current treatments for Alzheimer's disease: cholinesterase inhibitors. J Clin Psychiatry. 2003;64(suppl 9):11-17.

154.   **A**   **He experienced intense fear in the elevator**

The diagnostic criteria for acute stress disorder include the experience of intense fear, helplessness or horror, and subjective sense of numbing. The disturbances usually last for a minimum of 2 days and a maximum of 4 weeks and occur within 4 weeks of the traumatic event. Hypervigilance and increased arousal are usually present.

The DSM –IV-TR Criterion A for Acute stress disorder includes the following description. The person has been exposed to a traumatic event in which both of the following were present:

1) The person experienced, witnessed, or was confronted with an event or events that involved actual or threatened death or serious injury, or threat to the physical integrity of self or others.
2) The person's response involved intense fear, helplessness or horror.

1. American Psychiatric Association, The Diagnostic and Statistical Manual of Mental Disorders, 4th edition, Text Revision, DSM-IV-TR, American Psychiatric Association, Washington DC. 2003:469-72.

155. **E** **Aripiprazole**

Except for aripiprazole all the mentioned atypical antipsychotic medications mentioned have been FDA-approved for the long term treatment of schizophrenia. The efficacy of aripoprazole in treating schizophrenia was established in short term (4 and 6 weeks) controlled inpatient studies. According to the 2004 edition of the Physician's Desk Reference (PDR), physicians prescribing it for extended periods should periodically evaluate its long term usefulness for the individual patient. At the time of writing this question, Bristol-Myers Squibb Company, the manufacturer of aripiprazole, is seeking the FDA approval of its efficacy of treating long term schizophrenia.

1. Physician Desk Reference, 58th edition, Thomson PDR, Montvale NJ. 2004:1034,2496.

156. **A** **Fluoxetine dose reduction**

Adjunctive treatment with bupropion or topiramate can be considered if weight gain persists. Fluoxetine switching needs to be considered if depression reemerges. Adjunctive treatment with a 5-HT 2C agonist is irrelevant at this time since fluoxetine possesses potent 5- HT 2C action.

Fluoxetine most commonly causes anorexia leading to weight loss in most patients. Some patients however gain weight while taking it. Weight gain results from the medication itself or from the improved appetite that accompany the improved mood. In general diet and regular exercise are first recommended prior to the addition of weight reducing pharmacological interventions.

1. Gabbard GO. Treatments of Psychiatric disorders, 3rd edition. American Psychiatric Publishing Inc. Washington DC. 2001:2161-3,2212-3.

Medtext Medical World, Inc.

157.   C   Cocaine related CVA's are due to vasospasm

Most of the patients with cocaine related CVA's are in their mid 30's. Infarction and hemorrhages occur equally and are caused by vasospasm of the cerebral blood vessels which are thought to be induced either by cocaine itself or secondary to increased catecholamine levels. Brain stem infarctions are less common than cerebral hemisphere strokes. Preexisting lesions were evident in only about half of the intracerebral hemorrhages.

1. Sadock BJ, Sadock V. Kaplan & Sadock's Comprehensive Textbook of Psychiatry, 7th edition. Lippincott, Williams & Wilkins, New York NY. 2000:1003-7.

2. Auer J, Berent R, Eber B. Cardiovascular complications of cocaine use. *New England Journal of Medicine.* 2001;345:(21)1575-6.

158.   E   All of the above

> Fosphenytoin
> Thiamine
> Lorazepam
> Pyridoxine

Fosphenytoin and lorazepam are used for the treatment of recurrent generalized seizures. Thiamine is used to restore its depletion secondary to the daily intake of alcohol. Pyridoxine (Vitamin B6) is the antidote for isoniazid toxicity, which could lead to intractable seizures unresponsive to standard antiepileptic medications. Isoniazid most probably was used in this case for pulmonary tuberculosis.

1. Hales RE, Yudofsky SC. Textbook of Clinical Psychiatry, 4th edition. American Psychiatric Publishing Inc. Washington DC. 2003:347-9.

2. Baxter P, Clarke A, Cross H, Harding B, Hicks E, Livingston J, Surtees R. Idiopathic catastrophic epileptic encephalopathy presenting with acute onset intractable status. *Seizure* 2003;12(6):379-87.

159.   **B**   **Separation anxiety occurs between 10 and 16 months**

According to Margaret Mahler the separation-individuation phase of development begins in the fourth or fifth month of life and is completed by age 3. The characteristic anxiety during this phase of development is stranger anxiety which occur between 5 and 10 months. .In contrast to stranger anxiety which can occur even when the infant is in the mother's arm; separation anxiety is seen between the age of 10 and 16 months and is precipitated by separation from the person to whom the infant is attached. Rapprochement occurs between the age of 16 and 24 months; during that phase the infant struggles between wanting to be soothed by the mother and in the same time not wanting to accept her help.

1. Sadock BJ, Sadock V. Kaplan & Sadock's Comprehensive Textbook of Psychiatry, 7th edition. Lippincott, Williams & Wilkins. New York NY. 2000:1162-3&2926-8.

160.   **B**   **Euphoria**

The prefrontal cortex contains three regions; the orbitofrontal, the dorsolateral and the medial. Lesions to each region produce distinct syndromes. Damage to the orbitofrontal region of the brain causes lability, euphoria, irritability, lack of remorse, impaired judgment. Patients are also distractible. Patients may display apathetic indifference and then suddenly explode into impulsive disinhibition. Impairments in problem solving ability, retention as well as an altered sense of spontaneity may also occur.

1. Sadock BJ, Sadock V. Kaplan & Sadock's Comprehensive Textbook of Psychiatry, 7th edition. Lippincott, Williams & Wilkins. New York NY. 2000:243,932.

2.Victor M, Ropper AH. Adams and Victor's Principles of Neurology, 7th edition. McGraw-Hill Companies Inc. New York NY. 2001:472-7.

Medtext Medical World, Inc.

161. **A** **Hypersexuality**

Hypermetamorphosis is the inability to recognize the emotional significance of visual stimuli with constant shifting of attention. The condition occurs as a result of bitemporal lobe injury similar to the Klüver-Busy syndrome which is the experimental bitemporal lobe ablation in monkeys. Additional features include hypersexuality, tendency to explore the environment with the mouth and hyperphagia. Placidity rather than aggression usually occur. Phobias do not usually occur.

1. Sadock BJ, Sadock V. Kaplan and Sadock's Comprehensive Textbook of Psychiatry, 7th edition. Lippincott, Williams & Wilikins, New York NY. 2000:240-1.

162. **D** **Lorenz's concept of imprinting**

Imprinting was the experiment conducted by Konrad Lorenz when he moved and the newly hatched duckling followed him and reacted to him as if he was their mother duck. Harry Harlow studied the concept of surrogate mother in the Rhesus monkeys, who chose a cloth covered surrogate mother as opposed to a wire mother even if the later provided food. Eric Kandel studied the snail *Aplysia californica* in which learning lead to alteration of synaptic connection. Ivan Petrovich Pavlov described experimental neurosis occurring in dogs when they were unable to master an experimental situation

1. Sadock BJ, Sadock V. Kaplan and Sadock's Comprehensive Textbook of Psychiatry, 7th edition. Lippincott, Williams & Wilikins, New York NY. 2000:89-90,559-60.

Medtext Medical World, Inc.

163. **A** He may experience "visual non-verbal" task deficits

Right hemisphere lesions leading to left hemiparesis are associated with severe deficits on visual non-verbal tasks (such as memory for objects and faces) then auditory tasks (such as digit span). Episodic memory is memory for specific events. Semantic memory is related to remembering specific facts (such as knowing the president of the USA). Recent memory is related to events that occurred over the past few hours or days. Right hemisphere lesions do not affect memory however if aphasia develops, difficulty may be experienced in responding to memory testing.

1.Richardson MP, Strange BA, Duncan JS, Dolan RJ. Preserved verbal memory function in left medial temporal pathology involves reorganization of function to right medial temporal lobe. *Neuroimage* 2003;Suppl 1:S 112-9.

2. Sadock BJ, Sadock V. Kaplan and Sadock's Comprehensive Textbook of Psychiatry, 7th edition. Lippincott, Williams & Wilikins, New York NY. 2000:236-7, 307-9,433,685-5.

164. **B** Displacement

Phobia according to dynamic psychiatry is considered an abnormal fear resulting from a conflict related to sexual excitation attached to an unconscious object. The fear is avoided by displacing the conflict onto an object that is outside the ego system. The defense mechanism of displacement transfers the emotion from the original idea to which it is attached to another idea or object.

1. Sadock BJ, Sadock V. Kaplan and Sadock's Comprehensive Textbook of Psychiatry, 7th edition. Lippincott, Williams & Wilikins, New York NY. 2000:586,1469-70.

165.   D   The presence of normal language development

Options A, B, C & E are all features of Autistic disorder. The presence of normal language development is associated with Asperger's disorder in which there is no delay in language or cognitive development. Its prevalence is not known and appears to be more common in males. Asperger's disorder is similar to Autistic disorder in terms of impaired social interactions, restricted pattern of repetitive, stereotyped behaviors, limited interests and activities.

1. Hales RE, Yudofsky SG. Textbook of Clinical Psychiatry, 4th edition. American Psychiatric Publishing Inc. Washington DC. 2003;901-3.

2. Fitzergerald M. Callous/unemotional traits and Asperger's syndrome. *J Am Acad Child Adolesc Psychiatry*. 2003;42(9):1011.

166.   E   Delirium agitation is reduced with midazolam

Midazolam has been successfully used in the treatment of agitation in delirium. Dementia is a risk factor for delirium, however not all dementia patients develop delirium. The incidence of delirium is surgical patients varies between 4% and 31%.While sedation can decrease agitation in delirious patients, ongoing sedation could lead to respiratory depression and worsening of confusion. The 1:1 observation and the utilization of a "sitter" could ease the anxiety of staff and family members and could be used as a mean reporting ongoing behavioral change.

1. Young CC, Prielipp RC. Benzodiazepines in the intensive care unit. *Crit Care Clin*. 2001;17(4):843-62.

2. Gabbard GO. Treatment of Psychiatric Disorders, 3rd edition. American Psychiatric Publishing Inc. Washington DC. 2001:436.

167.   **B**   **Lewy Bodies are present in 25% of dementia cases**

Postmortem studies have revealed the presence of Lewy bodies in up to 25% of dementia cases. Vascular dementia accounts for 20% of cases. The mutation of chromosomes account for fewer than 5% of DAT. Neurofibrillary tangles are intracellular filaments, while the senile plaques are extracellular and contain beta amyloid. The early onset of the dementia of the Alzheimer's type is usually associated with rapid progression and deterioration.

1. Sadock BJ, Sadock V. Kaplan & Sadock's Comprehensive Textbook of Psychiatry, 7th edition. Lippincott, Williams & Wilkins. New York NY. 2000:287-8.

2.Rowland LP. Merritt's Neurology, 10[th]edition. Lippincott, Williams & Wilkins, Philadelphia PA. 2000:637-8.

168.   **A**   **Comorbid ADHD**

Individuals with Williams' syndrome present with elfin like faces, shirt status depressed nasal bridge, widely spaced teeth, a Starburst iris, renal and cardiovascular abnormalities supravalvular aortic stenosis, hypertension Thyroid abnormalities, hypercalcemia and a loquacious communication style known as "cocktail party speech". Comorbidities include ADHD, depression and anxiety. Williams syndrome occurs in 1/20,000 births, it is related to hemizygous deletion that includes elastin locus chromosome 7q11-23; autosomal dominant.

1. Sadock BJ, Sadock V. Kaplan & Sadock's Comprehensive Textbook of Psychiatry, 7th edition. Lippincott, Williams & Wilkins. New York NY. 2000:2596.

2. Sadock BJ, Sadock VA Kaplan & Sadock's Synopsis of Psychiatry, 9th edition. Lippincott Williams & Wilkins. Philadelphia PA. 2003:1171.

       Medtext Medical World, Inc.

169.   **E**   **The heart is among the target organ**

The tick-borne spirochetal infection is Lyme disease caused by the tick *Ixodes scapularis* which transfer the organism Borrelia burgdorferi causing initially flu-like syndrome and a rash taking place over days to weeks. Diagnosis may require several tests including Lyme ELISA(enzyme-linked immunosorbent assay) and Lyme Western blot and polymerace chain reaction assay (PCR).Even with early aggressive antibiotic treatment ,symptoms may recur or develop months to years later. Mood lability could develop as a complication of chronic encephalopathy. The organism can be lodged in its target organs which include the heart, eye, joint, muscles, and the nerves where it may lie dormant for months to years.

1. Wilson ME. Prevention of tick-borne diseases. *Med Clin North Am.* 2002;86(2):219-38.

2. Sadock BJ, Sadock V. Kaplan & Sadock's Comprehensive Textbook of Psychiatry, 7ᵗʰ edition. Lippincott, Williams & Wilkins. New York NY. 2000:336-9.

170.   **A**   **Motor aprosodia is present**

Motor aprosodia is the inability to affectively modulate speech and gestures. Sensory aprosodia is the inability to interpret the emotional components of other's speech or gestures. The aprosodic patient often appears emotionally blunted with flat affect. However this is a disorder of expression not a mood disorder and need to be differentiated from depression. Aprosodia usually follow right non-dominant hemisphere vascular insult.

1. Rowland LP. Merritt's Neurology, 10ᵗʰ edition. Lippincott, Williams & Wilkins. Philadelphia PA. 2000:680.

2. Mesulam MM. Primary progressive aphasia-a language-based dementia. *N Engl J Med.* 2003;349(16):1535-42.

Medtext Medical World, Inc.

171.   C   Release of dopamine

The positive reinforcement of alcohol appears to be mediated by activation of Gam aminobutyric acid -A (GABA-A) receptor, the release of opioid peptides and dopamine, the inhibition of glutamate and an interaction with serotonin systems. Many people use alcohol for its efficacy in alleviating anxiety. Perhaps 25 to 50 percent of patients with alcohol-related disorders also have co-morbid anxiety disorder especially those with phobias and panic disorder.

Alcohol may be used in an attempt to decrease symptoms of agoraphobia, or social phobia. Alcohol-related disorder is likely to precede the development of panic disorder or generalized anxiety disorder.

1. Sadock BJ, Sadock V. Kaplan & Sadock's Comprehensive Textbook of Psychiatry, 7th edition. Lippincott, Williams & Wilkins. New York NY. 2000:955-8.

172.   C   Joseph Wolpe: Behavior Therapy

Anna Freud is associated with ego psychology, while Heinz Kohut is associated with self-Psychology. Joseph Wolpe published the first book on behavior therapy. Donald Winnicott together with Melanie Klein is associated with object relationship theory. Isaac Mark demonstrated the effectiveness of behavioral therapy in treating social phobia. Interpersonal psychotherapy is credited to Gerald Klerman. Psychodynamic psychotherapy is based on psychoanalytic psychotherapy.

1. Kaplan BJ, Sadock V. Kaplan & Sadock's Comprehensive Textbook of Psychiatry, 7th edition. Lippincott, Williams & Wilkins. New York NY. 2000:3322.

Medtext Medical World, Inc.

173.   A   Bulimia Nervosa

It appears that two types of clinical disorders respond best to hypnosis. Disorders associated with the autonomic nervous system (anxiety, pain syndromes, irritable bowl syndrome and asthma) and those related to the principles of classical conditioning (phobias, nausea, vomiting and bulimia).

Most patients with uncomplicated bulimia nervosa do not require hospitalization, and they are not secretive about their illness.   However in some cases when eating binges are uncontrollable, or when additional psychiatric conditions exist with the emergence of suicidal intention, hospitalization becomes necessary. The combination of both psychotherapy and psychopharmacology with antidepressants has been effective particularly for binge purge cycles that do not respond to psychotherapy alone.

Classical conditioning, also called respondent conditioning, is the product of repeated pairing of neutral (conditioned stimulus); with one that evokes a response (unconditioned stimulus).   So the neutral stimulus (food) eventually evokes the response (eating and purging).   The extinction occurs when the conditioned stimulus is constantly repeated without the unconditioned stimulus.

1. Gabbard GO. Treatment of Psychiatric Disorders, 3rd edition. American Psychiatric Publishing Inc. Washington DC. 2001:2103-28.

2. Mantle F. Eating disorders: the role of hypnosis. *Paediatr Nurs.* 2003;15(7):42-5.

174.   C   Utilitarian-oriented position

Organ transplantation includes ethical and medical considerations. Pediatric candidates awaiting kidney transplant are given special priority due to potential growth delays associated with dialysis. Patients with psychiatric conditions including acute psychosis, active suicidal or homicidal ideations, current substance abusers, patients with dementia are all contraindications for organ transplants. Ventilator-dependent patients are excluded from lung transplants. Medical urgency does not override transplant recipient waiting list.

1. Kaplan BJ, Sadock V. Kaplan & Sadock's Comprehensive Textbook of Psychiatry, 7th edition. Lippincott, Williams & Wilkins. New York NY. 2000:3292-4.

2. Steiner RW .Consequences of selling a kidney in India. *JAMA*. 2003;289(6):698-9.

175.   E   All of the above

> Death will cause suffocation
> Death will bring intense guilt
> Death will cause intense pain
> Death will result in abandonment

Anxiety frequently arises or worsens toward the end of life. All the mentioned options are common and are not just limited to the patient but occur with family members, care givers and friends of the person facing death. Death is a universal unavoidable phenomenon. It arouses feelings of fear and dread in dying persons. Death may be considered as the absolute cessation of vital functions, and dying is the process of losing these functions. A terminally ill patient may not be afraid of death but he or she is terrified of the process of dying because it may be associated with abandonment, suffocation, pain and guilt over an unfulfilled life.

1. Kubler-Ross E. On Death and Dying. Macmillan, New York NY. 1969

2. Garros D, Rosychuck RJ, Cox PN. Circumstances Surrounding end of life in a pediatric intensive care unit. *Pediatrics*. 2003;112(5):e371.

176.   **D**   Magnetic gait

The features described are manifestations of normal pressure hydrocephalus (NPH) which is characterized by magnetic gait, urinary incontinence, dementia and improvement in cognition following serial lumbar punctures. NPH may follow a head injury, or an infection such as encephalitis. It is one of the treatable causes of dementia. In NPH the intra-cranial pressure is not acutely increased but is stable at the upper end of the normal range. Relief of the increased cerebrospinal fluid pressure may completely restore normal gait and cognitive functions.

1 .Victor M, Ropper AH. Adams and Victor's Principles of Neurology, 7th edition. McGraw-Hill Companies Inc. New York NY 2001:128.

2. Serot JM, Bene MC, Faure GC. Normal-pressure hydrocephalus and Alzheimer disease. *J Neuosurg.* 2003;99(4):797-8.

177.   **D**   Anhedonia

In addition to memory impairment all of the options may provide evidence for the diagnosis of DAT except for anhedonia which may suggest the presence of co-morbid depression. Anhedonia is the loss of interest in, and withdrawal from, all regular and pleasurable activities. It is usually associated with depression and is not a diagnostic criterion for DAT. Apathy is a state of dulled emotional tone, detachment and indifference and is associated with DAT.

1. American Psychiatric Association. The Diagnostic and Statistical Manual of Mental Disorders, 4th edition. Text Revision, DSM-IV-TR, American Psychiatric Association. Washington DC. 2000:147-67.

2. Sadock BJ, Sadock VA, Kaplan and Sadock's Synopsis of Psychiatry, 9th edition, Lippincott, Williams & Wilkins. Philadelphia PA. 2003:280-281.

178.   **D**   **Anticonvulsive agents**

Anticonvulsives with mood stabilizing properties may be useful in treating the described patient. Although antidepressants, especially the SSRI's, could be useful in treating impulse control disorders, the antidepressant mirtazapine has sedating properties but have not been studied in these conditions. There is no evidence to substantiate options A, B or E, in treating the conditions described. Pharmacotherapy in antisocial personality disorder may be useful in treating symptoms of rage, anxiety and depression; however the presence of substance abuse requires a judicial use of such interventions. Anticonvulsive agents such as carbamazepine and valproate can control impulsive behaviors especially if an EEG shows abnormal waveforms.

1. Hales RE, Yudofsky SC. Textbook of Clinical Psychiatry, 4th edition. American Psychiatric Publishing Inc. Washington DC. 2003:1110-4.

2. Koran LM, Chuong HW, Bullock KD, Smith SC. Citalopram for compulsive shopping disorder: an open-label study followed by double-blind discontinuation. *J Clin Psychiatry*. 2003;64(7):793-8.

179.   **B**   **Myoclonus**

The described symptoms suggest the development of "serotonin syndrome" brought on by taking serotonergic compounds such as citalopram, amitriptyline and St. John's Wort. It is characterized by myoclonus, fever, hypertension, confusion and tachycardia.

Concurrent administration of SSRI's or an SSRI with an MAOI, L-tryptophan or lithium can raise plasma serotonin concentrations to toxic levels, producing several symptoms called *serotonin syndrome*. It is a potentially serious syndrome and can lead to delirium, coma, status epilepticus, cardiovascular collapse and death. Treatment consists of removing the offending agents and promptly instituting supportive intense medical treatment with nitroglycerin, cyproheptadine, methysergide, cooling blankets, dantrolene, anticonvulsants, benzodiazepines and mechanical ventilation.

1. Hales RE, Yudofsky SC. Textbook of Clinical Psychiatry, 4th edition. American Psychiatric Publishing Inc. Washington DC. 2003:1059.

2. Garside S, Rosebush PI. Serotonin syndrome: not a benign toxidrome. *CMAJ* 2003;169(6):543.

180.   **E**   **Single bedtime lowest effective dose is recommended**

Polyuria occurs in up to 70% of patients on lithium maintenance therapy. Thiazide diuretics markedly reduce urine volume caused by nephrogenic DI. To develop nephrogenic DI urine output should be greater than 3 L/day. Nephrogenic DI is diagnosed in 10% of lithium treated patients. The polyuria results from lithium antagonism to the effects of the antidiuretic hormone, which then causes diuresis. If nephrogenic DI develops, the renal function should be evaluated and followed up with 24-hour urine collection for creatinine clearance determinations. Treatment consists of fluid replacement, the use of the lowest effective lithium dosage, and single daily dosing.

1. Gabbard GO. Treatment of Psychiatric Disorders, 3rd edition. American Psychiatric Publishing Inc. Washington DC. 2001:1170

181.   **E**   **Hypochondriasis**

The belief of being ill rather than having a specific illness is one of the core criterions of diagnosing hypochondriasis. The symptoms are not intentionally produced as in factitious disorder. There is no description of symptoms to suggest histrionic personality or somatization disorder. In somatic delusions the belief of being ill is unshakable. Since the treatment of hypochondriasis and somatic delusional disorder are completely different it is of paramount importance to make an accurate diagnosis of hypochondriasis.

1. American Psychiatric Association. The Diagnostic and Statistical Manual of Mental Disorders, 4th edition. Text Revision, DSM-IV-TR, American Psychiatric Association. Washington DC. 2000:504-7.

2. Khouzam HR, Field S. Somatization disorder: clinical presentation and treatment in primary care. *Hospital Physician.* 1999;35(4):20-4.

182.   **D**   **Increased sexual excitement**

The acute effects of (crack) cocaine include vasoconstriction, increased heart rate, increased blood pressure, euphoria with increased energy, heightened alertness, increased anxiety, decreased appetite and increased sexual excitement. Crack is a free base form of cocaine. It is extremely potent and usually sold in small, ready-to-smoke amounts often called "rocks". Crack is highly addictive; even after one or two experiences with it, intense craving develops. Although cocaine is used as an aphrodisiac and as a mean to delay sexual orgasm, its repeated use can result in impotence.

1.Sadock BJ, Sadock V. Kaplan and Sadock's Comprehensive Textbook of Psychiatry, 7th edition. Lippincott Williams & Wilkins. New York NY. 2000:1006-7.

2.Khouzam HR. Helping your patients beat cocaine addiction. The four dimensions of treatment. *Postgraduate Medicine.* 1999;105(3):185-91.

183.   **C**   **Fragile X Syndrome**

The three most common cause of mental retardation (MR) that account for 30% of identified cases are Down's syndrome, fragile X-syndrome and fetal alcohol syndrome.

Copraxia and stereotype are some of the behavioral manifestations of MR. Prader-Willis syndrome is not considered a common cause of MR, its associated features include short stature, obesity, hypogonadism and hyperphagia.

Williams syndrome is associated with anxiety, hyperactivity, fears and higher verbal than visual spatial skills.

Fragile X Syndrome has an extremely high rate of attention deficit hyperactivity disorder and a high rate of aberrant interpersonal and language functions. It often meets the criteria for autistic disorder and avoidant personality disorder.

1. Sadock BJ,Sadock V. Kaplan and Sadock's Comprehensive Textbook of Psychiatry, 7th edition. Lippincott Williams & Wilkins. New York NY. 2000:2593-9.

2. Hassink S. Problems in childhood obesity. *Prim Care.* 2003;30(2):357-74.

184. **B** **Subthalamic nucleus**

Electrodes with high-frequency stimulation of the subthalamic nucleus, has produced impressive improvement in all features of Parkinson's disease. Transcranial magnetic stimulation (TMS) involves a strong electromagnet, in which the field is oscillated at various frequencies, pulse duration and intensity. When TMS is given as a train of pulses aimed at specific regions of the basal ganglia and the subthalamic nucleus, it can eliminate the tremor of Parkinson's disease.

1. Victor M, Ropper AH. Adams and Victor's Principles of Neurology, 7th edition. Mc Graw-Hill Companies Inc. New York NY. 2001:1136-7.

2. Ondo W, Almaguer M, Jankovic J, Simpson RK. Thalamic deep brain stimulation: comparison between unilateral and bilateral placement. *Arch Neurol.* 2001;58(2):218-27.

185. **A** **Physostigmine**

The most serious effect of anticholinergic toxicity is anticholinergic intoxication. It is characterized by delirium, seizures, hallucinations, agitation and coma. Flushing, mydriasis, dry mouth, hypertension and decreased bowel sounds also can occur. In general physostigmine should only be used to confirm the diagnosis of anticholinergic activity or for the treatment of anticholinergic intoxication.

The adverse effects of anticholinergic drugs result from the blockade of muscarinic acetylcholine receptors. The most serious symptoms of anticholinergic intoxication are seizures, severe hypertension and delirium. Physostigmine is an inhibitor of anticholinesterase and is given 1 to 2 mg I.V. (1 mg every 2 minutes) or I.M. (every 30-60 minutes). This can only be used with the presence of emergency cardiac monitoring and life support services. Physostigmine can precipitate severe hypotension and bronchial constriction, and it is contraindicated in patients with unstable vital signs, asthma or a history of cardiac abnormalities. The adverse effects of physostigmine can be reversed by the rapid administration of intramuscular atropine.

1. Sadock BJ, Sadock V. Kaplan and Sadock's Comprehensive Textbook of Psychiatry, 7th edition. Lippincott Williams & Wilkins. New York NY. 2000:2350.

186. **D** **Designed for diseases with low incidence**

A case-control study is a retrospective study that examines persons with very rare diseases. It is appropriate in answering epidemiological questions related to diseases with low incidence rate. Epidemiological studies in psychiatry are mostly experimental due to the difficulties with finding control subjects. The design of experimental studies attempts to answer questions about the etiology, treatment, course, prognosis and prevention of various psychiatric disorders. Prospective studies also called "longitudinal studies" are based on observing events as they occur. Retrospective studies are based on analyzing past data or past events. Case-history study is a retrospective study that examines patients with a particular disease. Cross-sectional studies provide information about the prevalence of diseases. They are also known as prevalence studies.

1. Sadock BJ, Sadock V. Kaplan and Sadock's Comprehensive Textbook of Psychiatry, 7th edition. Lippincott Willims & Wilkins. New York NY. 2000:509-10.

187. **D** **Citalopram**

Among all the mentioned SSRI's antidepressants citalopram has a very low to no inhibition of the P-450 isoenzyme systems. Most psychotherapeutic drugs are oxidized by the hepatic cytochrome P450 (CYP) enzyme system which is so named based on its strong absorption of light at a wave length of 450 mm. The SSRI's have a number of pharmacokinetic interactions with the CYP enzyme system and citalopram is not considered as a potent inhibitor of the CYP enzyme system.

1. Gabbard GO. Treatment of Psychiatric Disorders, 3rd edition. American Psychiatric Publishing Inc. Washington DC. 2001:1391

188. **C** **Establishment of a psychotherapeutic focus**

Short-term dynamic psychotherapy as conducted by Habib Davanlo at McGill University, requires candidates with psychological mindedness, flexible defense mechanisms, who have at least one past meaningful relationship and its goal is to establish a therapeutic focus. Patients undergoing short-term dynamic psychotherapy need to be able to tolerate affect, as well as be able to show good response to trial transference interpretations. The patients need to have a high level of motivation and lack the defense mechanisms of projection, splitting and denial. Although short-term dynamic psychotherapy has no specific termination date and patients are told that treatment will be short. Longer durations are also allowed for seriously ill patients.

1. Sadock BJ, Sadock V. Kaplan and Sadock's Comprehensive Textbook of Psychiatry, 7th edition. Lippincott Williams & Wilkins. New York NY. 2000:2072-75.

2. Gabbard GO. Treatment of Psychiatric Disorders, 3rd edition. American Psychiatric Publishing Inc. Washington DC. 2001:831-3.

189.   D   Obsessive-compulsive disorder

Group A beta-hemolytic streptococcus infection has been associated with either initial onset or an exacerbation of obsessive compulsive disorder (OCD) in children and adolescents. Interests have been established in relation to the possible link between group A beta hemolytic streptococcal infection and OCD. This type of infection can cause rheumatic fever, Sydenham's chorea and show OCD symptoms of recurrent and distressing ideas (obsessions) that are intrusive in one's thoughts. These may lead to repetitive and purposeful behaviors (compulsions). It is not clear if the treatment of the beta A hemolytic streptococcus would lead to the permanent remission of these OCD symptoms.

1. Gabbay V, Coffey B. Obsessive-Compulsive Disorder, Tourette's Disorder, or Pediatric Autoimmune Neuropsychiatric Disorders Associated with Streptococcus in an Adolescent? Diagnostic and Therapeutic Challenges. J Child Adolesc Psychopharmacol. 2003;13(3):209-12.

2. Sadock BJ, Sadock V. Kaplan and Sadock's Comprehensive Textbook of Psychiatry, 7th edition. Lippincott Willims & Wilkins. New York NY. 2000:1456.

190.   D   Projection

Projection is a narcissistic defense mechanism in which the individual perceives and reacts to unacceptable inner impulses as though they are outside his/her own self. According to Sigmund Freud, the founder of classic psychoanalysis, each phase of libidinal development, evokes characteristic ego defenses. These defense mechanisms can be grouped according to the relative degree of maturity associated with them. Projection is one of the narcissistic defenses. Narcissistic defenses are the most primitive and appear in children and in people with psychosis and include both perception of one's own feelings in another and subsequent acting on the perception (psychotic paranoid delusions). On a psychotic level, the defense mechanism of projection takes the form of frank delusions about external reality (usually persecutory).

1. Sadock BJ, Sadock V. Kaplan and Sadock's Comprehensive Textbook of Psychiatry, 7th edition. Lippincott Willims & Wilkins. New York NY. 2000:1731.

191.   D   Alcohol

Asians may develop an idiosyncratic physiologic reaction. This reaction is a manifestation of early onset of toxic symptoms of alcohol intoxication. It has been attributed to the decreased function of alcohol-metabolizing enzymes in Asian people. Alcohol is metabolized by two enzymes: alcohol dehydrogenase (ADH) and aldehyde dehydrogenase. ADH catalyzes the conversion of alcohol into acetaldehyde, which is a toxic compound. Aldehyde dehydrogenase catalyzes the conversion of acetaldehyde into acetic acid. The decreased function of alcohol-metabolizing enzymes in some Asian people can lead to an easy alcohol intoxication and alcohol toxic symptoms.

1. Sadock BJ, Sadock V. Kaplan and Sadock's Comprehensive Textbook of Psychiatry, 7th edition. Lippincott Williams & Wilkins. New York NY. 2000:956.

192.   **A**   **Superoxide dismutase (SOD)**

Superoxide dismutase has been implicated as a gene mutation in ALS, LIM kinase-1gene is related to a gene mutation in Williams' syndrome, Beta-globin is a gene related to sickle cell anemia, tau and beta amyloid protein are related to possible gene mutation in Alzheimer's disease. ALS begins in adult life and progresses over months or years to involve all the striated muscles (including those involved in chewing and swallowing). ALS spares the cardiac and ocular muscles. In addition to muscle atrophy, patients with ALS may have signs of pyramidal tract involvement. This is a rapid progressing disease and death generally occurs within 4 years of onset.

1.Victor M, Ropper AH. Adams and Victor's Principles of Neurology, 7th edition, McGraw-Hill Companies Inc, New York NY. 2001:1157

2.Sadock BJ, Sadock VA. Kaplan and Sadock's Synopsis of Psychiatry Behavioral Sciences /Clinical Psychiatry, 9th edition. Lippincott Williams & Wilkins. Philadelphia PA. 2003:122-8.

193.   **B**   **Dialectical therapy**

This type of therapy was developed by M. Lineham as a training manual to treat BPD. It combines aspects of cognitive and behavior therapy. It has been effective in diminishing suicidal acts that are often associated with BPD.

Dialectical behavior therapy (DBT) has five essential "functions" in treatment.

1) Enhance and expand the repertoire of skillful behavioral patterns
2) Improve motivation to change by reducing reinforcement of maladaptive behaviors
3) Ensure that newly acquired behavioral patterns are generalized from the therapeutic setting to the natural environment
4) Structure the environment so that effective behaviors are reinforced
5) Enhance the motivation and skills of the therapist so that effective treatment is rendered to BPD patients

1. Gabbard GO. Treatment of Psychiatric Disorders, 3rd edition. American Psychiatric Publishing Inc. Washington DC. 2001:2279-80.

Medtext Medical World, Inc.

194.   D   Early age of onset

Early age of onset in the absence of precipitating events with a family history of schizophrenia, insidious onset, poor premorbid functioning, poor support systems, predominance of negative symptoms, presence of neurological signs and symptoms, history of head trauma and the presence of expressed emotions, all have been associated with poor prognosis in schizophrenia. Expressed emotions is a term used to describe families that display excessive hostility, anxiety, over-concern, or over-protectiveness toward patients with schizophrenia leading to risk of relapse into psychosis. Genetic studies of schizophrenia show that a person is likely to have schizophrenia when other members of the family have the disorder and the correlation depends on the closeness of the familial relationship. Monozygotic twins have the highest concordance rate. Twins raised by adoptive parents have the same rate of schizophrenia as their siblings brought up by their biological parents.

1. Hales RE, Yudofsky SC. Textbook of Clinical Psychiatry, 4th edition. American Psychiatric Publishing Inc. Washington DC. 2003:400.

195.   A   A resting tremor

Parkinson's disease (PD) symptoms include a tremor in a resting position, which is inhibited by volitional movements. PD is characterized by the triad of resting tremor, rigidity and bradykinesia. The resting tremor is a coarse, rhythmic, with a frequency of 3 to 6 cycles per second, affecting the limbs, hand, mouth or tongue. Rigidity is characterized by muscular "cogwheel" or continuous "lead pipe" rigidity. Bradykinesia includes the mask–like facial appearance, decreased accessory arm movements during walking and a characteristic difficulty in initiating movements. Other PD is also associated with features of slowed thinking, excessive salivation, drooling, shuffling gait, micrographia, seborrhea, dysphoric mood and depression

1. Bradley WG, Daroff RB, Fenichel GM, Marsden CD. Neurology in Clinical Practice, 3rd edition. Butterworth-Heinemann, Boston MA. 2000:1892-3.

196.   D   Nortriptyline

The tricyclic antidepressant nortriptyline has been used to treat diabetic peripheral neuropathy. Its therapeutic effects can be measured with blood level monitoring since it possesses a 50-150 ng/mL therapeutic window. The tricyclic antidepressants amitriptyline and nortriptyline and the SSRI sertraline have been used to alleviate the pain of peripheral neuropathy. Whether this is an antidepressant effect or an independent analgesic effect is still undetermined. However this pain reducing effect supports the hypothesis that serotonin is important in the pathophysiology of pain.

When nortriptyline is used as an antidepressant its response rate decreases if it is either below or above the therapeutic window. The clinical relevance of the therapeutic window in managing peripheral neuropathy has not yet been established. Antidepressant blood monitoring is not routinely used except for monitoring of compliance and/or adverse effects.

1. Sadock BJ, Sadock V. Kaplan and Sadock's Comprehensive Textbook of Psychiatry, 7th edition. Lippincott Williams & Wilkins. New York NY. 2000:745.

197.   E   None of the above

According to the NIMH-ECA, the lifetime rates of antisocial personality disorders have been equal in African Americans, Hispanics, Caucasian non-Hispanics and Asians. The NIMH-ECA study used diagnostic tools with more specific criteria to make reliable diagnosis of the percentage of the population with mental disorders. Various sites around the country were selected to assess mental disorder prevalence, incidence, and service use in geographically defined community populations of at least 200,000 residents. The NIMH-ECA project evolved from the report of the 1977 President's Commission on Mental Health, which highlighted the need to identify the mentally ill and indicate how they are treated and by whom.

1. Sadock BJ, Sadock V. Kaplan and Sadock's Comprehensive Textbook of Psychiatry, 7th edition. Lippincott Williams & Wilkins. New York NY. 2000:519.

2. Regier DA, Farmer ME, Rae DS, Locke BZ, Keith SJ, Judd LL, Goodwin FK. Comorbidity of mental disorders with alcohol and other drug abuse. Results from the Epidemiologic Catchment Area (ECA). *JAMA* (see comments)1990;264(19):2511-8.

198.   **B**   **Abstract reasoning**

The Wisconsin Card Sorting Test (WCST) assesses abstract reasoning and flexibility in problem solving. Abnormal responses appeared in people with damage to their frontal lobes and the caudate, also in patients with MS and in schizophrenia. The WCST consists of stimulus cards of different color, form and number that are presented to patients to sort into groups according to a principle established by the examiner but unknown to the patient. The correct and incorrect responses are conveyed to the patient and then the number of trials to achieve 10 consecutive correct responses is calculated. When the process is repeated several times, it measures the capacity for abstract thinking (i.e. the number of trials required to achieve a solution) and flexibility (preservative errors on successive sorting trials).

1. Sadock BJ, Sadock V. Kaplan and Sadock's Comprehensive Textbook of Psychiatry, 7th edition. Lippincott Williams & Wilkins. New York NY. 2000:304.

2. Sadock BJ, Sadock VA Kaplan and Sadock's Synopsis of Psychiatry,9th edition. Lippincott, Williams & Wilkins. Philadelphia PA. 2003:186.

199.   **D**   **Unfavorable**

In general, an unfavorable prognosis in multiple sclerosis (M.S.) is associated with a late onset, progressive course from onset, male sex, poor recovery from exacerbations, and early cerebellar involvement. Increasingly patients with these somewhat guarded-to-grim risk factors are reasonably aware of their somewhat dismal prognoses and are somewhat assisted by support groups. A positive outlook on the part of both caregivers and healthcare providers may prove both empowering and helpful. Patient education may reasonably well correlate with patient compliance with the ongoing therapy teams and support systems to assist the patient with activities of daily living (A.D.L.).

1. Kos K. and Cross A., "Understanding Multiple Sclerosis," Emergency Medicine, 2001:60. www.emedmag.com

200.   **E**   **All of the above**

> Problems with concentration
> Problems with attention
> Problems with recent memory
> Problems with information processing

Neurological testing has demonstrated and documented the extent of cognitive impairment in 70% of multiple sclerosis (M.S.) patients. Current therapy appears to be limited to slowing of the cognitive deterioration with the beta interferon agents. Recognition of cognitive impairment in patients with multiple sclerosis may well be an important insight into meeting the needs of patients with multiple sclerosis and meeting the needs of their caregivers as well.

1. Kos K. and Cross A., "Understanding Multiple Sclerosis," Emergency Medicine, 2001:60. www.emedmag.com

201.   **B**   **Levodopa**

Levodopa is the metabolic precursor of dopamine that has proven to be helpful to the second most common neurodegenerative disorder known as Parkinson's Disorder. Lidocaine may be provided in ventricular tachyarrhythmias. Lithium may be provided in mania. Lamivudine may be provided in the treatment of the acquired immune deficiency syndrome (A.I.D.S.).

1. Clinical Update, Emergency Medicine, "Pramipexole in the Treatment of Early Parkinson's Disease," 2001:31

202.   **E**   **90%**

Ninety percent of patients taking levodopa experience dyskinesia and or hallucinations. The newer non-ergoline, dopaminergic agonist pramipexole has been shown to be safe and effective in Parkinson's Disorder. On the one hand, the Parkinson's Study Group (an independent consortium of investigators) in a double-blinded clinical trial comparing pramipexole with levodopa showed that the risk of motor complications in patients taking pramipexole is 55% lower than among patients receiving levodopa. On the other hand,

Medtext Medical World, Inc.

levodopa is generally more effective in reducing the severity of Parkinson's Disorder. Finally the Quality-of-Life scores at 23.5 months were higher in patients in the levodopa group than in the pramipexole group.

1. Clinical Update, Emergency Medicine, "Pramipexole in the Treatment of Early Parkinson's Disease," 2001:31

203.   A   Basophilic stippling of her red blood cells

Magnetic resonance imaging (M.R.I.), computerized axial tomography (C.T.) scan, electroencephalography (E.E.G.), and electromyography (E.M.G.) are time-consuming, costly tests. Microscopic examination of Susan's red blood cells revealed, "basophilic stippling;" a clue to her (herbal-induced) lead poisoning. Susan's blood lead level was 86mg/dL Susan's urine lead level was 150mg/dL. After treatment, Susan was able to provide the additional history that she had, "Increased her herbal supplements when she began to drop basketballs (clumsiness of her hands), and she began to stumble (foot drop) on the basketball court."

1. Ewer M.S., "Case of the Month," Internal Medicine World Report, 2001:7

204.   C   Sam and Marsha

The highest driver fatality rates are found in the youngest and oldest drivers. The risk of a fatal crash increases with increasing blood alcohol level. Elevating the minimum legal drinking age to 21 has resulted in significant decreases in traffic crashes and fatalities. Lowering the legal blood alcohol level limit for adult drivers to 0.08 percent is associated with decreased alcohol related fatal crashes. License confiscation at the time of arrest reduces alcohol-related fatal crashes and repeated Driving under the Influence (D.U.I.) offenses.

1. Gordis E., "Alcohol Alert: National Institute on Alcohol Abuse and Alcoholism," Number 52, 2001:1

205.   **C**   **30%**

Meningiomas account for 30% of the incidental tumors found at autopsy. In other words, in 30% of the post mortem examinations, the deceased has died with the meningioma but not of the meningioma. These data may well underscore and emphasize the importance and value of performing post mortem examinations in the general population, if for no other reason or purpose, than to ascertain the genetic burden of malignancy among the surviving family of the deceased.

1. Kostandy G. et. al, "Intracranial Meningiomas: A Clinical Update," Resident & Staff Physician, 2001:35

206.   **D**   **Jill**

While a meningioma can occur at virtually any age and is well described as an incidental finding at autopsy (post mortem examination); nevertheless, the percentage of meningiomas found in the general patient population increases with age. The female to male ratio of intracranial meningiomas found in the general patient population is (2:1). Can we use these percentages to sharpen our diagnostic skills by raising the level of our index of suspicion of meningioma in our senior citizens in general and in our senior women citizens in particular?

1. Kostandy G. et. al, "Intracranial Meningiomas: A Clinical Update," Resident & Staff Physician, 2001:35

207.   **A**   **Sphenoidal wing**

Visual impairment, facial pain and anesthesia are consistent with fifth cranial nerve damage, associated with cranial nerve (3rd, 4th, and 6th) palsy implicates the sphenoidal wing. Parasagittal involvement would be present with partial seizures and leg weakness. Olfactory groove involvement would present with loss of sense of smell (anosmia) and reduced intellectual functioning (dementia). Suprasellar tumors would present with a bitemporal hemianopsia. Infratentorial tumors would present with headache, vertigo and ataxia.

1. Kostandy G. et. al, "Intracranial Meningiomas: A Clinical Update," Resident & Staff Physician, 2001:47

208.   **C**   **Predominantly benign but may be atypically malignant**

Although meningiomas are histopathologically predominantly benign tumors, invasion of both dura matter and cranial bone may occur. Complete surgical removal can be difficult. Recurrence rates range from 10% in histopathologically benign meningiomas to 90% in atypical malignant meningiomas. Patients with surgically resected meningiomas may need to be followed with either magnetic resonance imaging (M.R.I.) with gadolinium or computerized axial tomography (C.A.T.) scanning with contrast media.

1. Kostandy G. et. al, "Intracranial Meningiomas: A Clinical Update," Resident & Staff Physician, 2001:47

209.   **E**   **All of the above**

Screaming
Throwing objects
Striking objects
Striking others

Survivors may also speak in a loud voice, and may strike objects with or without a specific target in mind. Survivors may also endorse verbal demands such as, "Where is the doctor," and may endorse verbal abuse such as, "You should have been able to save him." The pain and suffering of the survivors may well have been defined by F. Scott Fitzgerald's writing that, "There are no scars on the soul...only open wounds..."

1. Iserson K.V., "The Gravest Words: Notifying, Survivors about Sudden, Unexpected Deaths," Resident & Staff Physician, 2001:66

210.   **E**   **All of the above**

God never gives us more than we can handle
Only the good die young
Aren't you lucky that at least you were married for six years with children?
You must be strong for your children

Both "God clichés" (A and B) and "Unhealthy expectations" (C and D) must be avoided. Other harmful phrases to be avoided include: "It was actually a blessing because... (God cliché)," "It must have been his time to go (Basic ignorance)," "Everything is going to be O.K., (Basic insensitivity)," Did he make peace with God before he died (Basic insensitivity)?

1. Iserson K.V., "The Gravest Words: Notifying, Survivors about Sudden, Unexpected Deaths," Resident & Staff Physician, 2001:66.

Medtext Medical World, Inc.

211. **E** **All of the above**

I cannot imagine how difficult this is for you
I know this is very painful for you
It is harder, much harder than most people think
It is O.K. to be angry with God

You may also endorse, "I'm so sorry for your loss," which is inclusive without pitying; and you may endorse, "It must be hard to accept." Non verbal communication can be improved by practicing facial gestures in front of a mirror may well give providers some idea how their facial gestures may be perceived by survivors. Your kind words and your nonjudgmental tone of voice and facial gestures resolve the crisis. Mary collapses sobbing into your arms. Keisha and Elijah are provided care by social services. Care is provided for the "kicked" hospital employees. The hospital Chaplain provides spiritual support for Mary. The police marksman stands down.

1. Iserson K.V., "The Gravest Words: Notifying, Survivors about Sudden, Unexpected Deaths," Resident & Staff Physician, 2001:66

212. **E** **Cellular phones are not associated with brain tumors**

Handheld cellular phones are not associated with the risk of brain cancer. While we concede that there may well be times that providers might consider leaving an issue within a gray area this is not one of those times. The issue is clear and need to be made crystal clear in a complete, concise, frank, factual response.

1. Muscat J.E. et. al.,"Handheld Cellular Telephone Use and Risk of Brain Cancer," Journal of the American Medical Association, 284:3001-7, 2000

213.　　**D**　　**Testosterone**

Counterintuitive those this issue may well be; nevertheless, androgens provide the basis for both sexual desire and sexual response in both men and women. Testosterone cypionate (Depo-Testosterone) monthly injections would be expected to improve Diane's sexual performance within 3 months. The selective serotonin reuptake inhibitors (S.S.R.I's); fluoxetine (Prozac), sertraline (Zoloft), and paroxetine (Paxil), would not be expected to improve Diane's sexual performance. Estrogen provided in the form of estradiol cypionate (Depo-Estradiol) would only be of value if Diane were symptomatic of estrogen deprivation.

1. Seifer, Judy A. Ph.D., R.N., "Reduced Libido in a Woman with Surgical Menopause," Medical Aspects of Human Sexuality, www.medicalsexuality.org July 10, 2001:1

214.　　**D**　　**Eflornithine hydrochloride (Vaniqa)**

The new preparation, eflornithine hydrochloride (Vaniqa) will remove Diane's facial hair that results when testosterone is metabolized to dihydrotestosterone which is the active hormone that stimulates hair growth. Vaniqa can spare Diane the skin irritation caused by depilatories and shaving; and, the time and expense of electrolysis. The application eflornithine hydrochloride (Vaniqa) with removal of Diane's facial hair may well be quintessential to Diane's self image, self-actualization, and self-fulfillment as a woman.

1. Seifer, Judy A. Ph.D., R.N., "Reduced Libido in a Woman with Surgical Menopause," Medical Aspects of Human Sexuality, www.medicalsexuality.org July 10, 2001:1

Medtext Medical World, Inc.

215. **E** **All of the above**

Most women are not consistently orgasmic with penile-vaginal intercourse
A program of directed masturbation has been shown to be effective for woman with female orgasmic disorder
Women exhibit great variability in the type and intensity of stimulation required to trigger an orgasm
Couple therapy that focuses on communication skills has been shown to be effective

A program of directed masturbation has been shown to be effective for woman with female orgasmic disorder. Women exhibit great variability in the type and intensity of stimulation required to trigger an orgasm Couple therapy that focuses on communication skills has been shown to be effective Making the time to provide psycho-educational sex therapy within the setting of couples and/or marital therapy will provide a reasonably positive approach to inhibited female orgasm also known as female orgasmic disorder. John needs to learn, although Jane probably already knows, that their two most important sex organs are their skin and their brain. Making the time to educate the couple to make time for themselves, for each other, for psychosexual activity, up to and including scheduling psychosexual activity on a calendar much as they might schedule any other event or issue in their lives may well enhance their joy in their marriage. Moreover reduction of performance pressure will have an increased probability of enhancing their marriage; for example, instructions to simply give each other a hug or a foot massage, and to go no further than that hug or that foot massage, may well have a high probability of restoring their focus on the pleasure of the moment thereby reducing their performance pressure to achieve orgasmic release!

1. Hales R.E. (Editor) "American Psychiatric Association Textbook of Psychiatry," Third Edition, American Psychiatric Association Press: Washington, D.C., 1999:750

216.   **C**   Uncertain if anti-depressants are unsafe for nursing mothers

The advantages of breast milk to infants in the first six months include reducing the neonatal incidence of:

1 Gastrointestinal disorders
2   Respiratory ailments
3 Anemia
4 Otitis media

As well as providing opportunity for infant-maternal bonding as there are no controlled studies on the safety of psychotropic medications in nursing mothers; this may well be a judgment call on the part of the psychiatrist; i.e., how many bouts of depression has Susan experienced and how severe were Susan's bouts of depression? It is reasonable to keep Susan's pediatrician fully informed to facilitate monitoring of her newborn, nursing infant.

1. Burt, Vivian K., M.D., Ph.D., et. al., Reviews and Overviews: "The Use of Psychotropic Medications during Breast-Feeding," American Journal of Psychiatry 158:7, July 2001:1001

217.   **B**   Magnetic Resonance Imaging

A T1-weighted sagital magnetic resonance imaging (M.R.I.) of Carla's brain revealed a mass in the inferior region of Carla's fourth ventricle. Her mass — a choroid-plexus tumor - caused Carla's vomiting by stimulation of her vomiting center in the dorsal portion of her lateral reticular formation and her chemoreceptor trigger zone in her area postrema of the floor of her fourth ventricle. Carla's choroid-plexus tumor was surgically removed and her vomiting stopped. Carla returned to her active military flying duty status.

1. Garcia-Monaco` J.C., and Larena J.A., Images in Clinical Medicine: "Vomiting of Neurologic Origin," New England Journal of Medicine, Volume 345, Number 01, 5 July 2001:33.

218.   **D**   **All of the above**

Ten years after heroin rehabilitation, 15% die
Twenty years after heroin rehabilitation, 30% die
Thirty years after heroin rehabilitation, 50% die

Despite the ongoing expenditure of vast sums of money and ongoing vast numbers of chemical dependency recovery providers and chemical dependency recovery programs, opiate dependence remains a chronic illness with a poor prognosis. The most common causes of death include:

1. Accidental poisoning
2. Drug overdose
3. Suicide
4. Homicide
5. Accidents
6. Chronic liver disease
7. Heart disease
8. Cancer

Our opiate dependent patients and their families need to be informed from their initial recovery period that their prognosis may well be guarded (poor). These efforts and endeavors to provide patient education and family and/or significant other education need to be documented in the chronological record of medical care. Verbalization of understanding of the patient and family education needs to be documented as well. Twelve step work with sponsorship in Narcotics Anonymous (N.A.) for our opiate dependent patients and in AL-anon for their families and/or significant others may well be helpful in assisting opiate dependent patients and their families to develop and use their Tools of Recovery.

1. "Opiate Dependence: A Chronic Illness with a Poor Prognosis," Archives of General Psychiatry," #58. 2001:503-508

219.   **B**   **20%**

When 240 heroin-dependent individuals were interviewed after a 30 year follow-up, 60% had negative urine tests for opiates, 20% were still using heroin, 10% refused to give urine specimens for drug screening, and another 10% were incarcerated in correctional facilities (jail or prison) and could not be tested. Twelve step work with sponsorship in Narcotics Anonymous for the opiate dependent patients and in AL-anon for their families and/or significant others may well be helpful in assisting opiate dependent patients and their families to develop and use their "Tools of Recovery."

1. "Opiate Dependence: A Chronic Illness with a Poor Prognosis," Archives of General Psychiatry, #58:.May 2001:503-508

220.   **E**   **50%**

The average period of continuous abstinence from heroin was ten years. Mortality is high. Cycles of abstinence and relapse are to be anticipated and expected. Only fifty percent of the studied heroin-dependent individuals were abstinent for more than 5 years. Twelve step work with sponsorship in Narcotics Anonymous or a related program for the opiate dependent patients and in AL-anon or a related program for the families and/or significant others may well be helpful in assisting opiate dependent patients and their families to develop and use their "Tools of Recovery" and is reasonably consistently associated with a sustained recovery.

1."Opiate Dependence: A Chronic Illness with a Poor Prognosis," Archives of General Psychiatry," #58: 2001:503-508.

Medtext Medical World, Inc.

221. **A** **Hippocampus**

When the researchers stimulated the "glutamate-rich" region of the hippocampus (which is an important area for memory), the rats began to "push the cocaine bar!" That the "glutamate-rich" region of the rat hippocampus is important in triggering drug-seeking behavior may well figure prominently in the problem of human chemical dependency. More basic research may well be needed to provide a more complete understanding of the pathophysiology (mechanism) of "craving" in general and "cocaine craving" in particular.

1. Science: #292 2001:1175-8

2. Science: #292 2001:1039

222. **C** **Bill**

Our psychiatric literature supports the statement that pathological gambling is a psychiatric disorder. As with any disorder, identifying those most at risk would appear to be a reasonable first step in providing treatment and care. Elderly men, of the so called "working class" appear to be most at risk of pathological gambling. Dare we inquire what role does our folklore play in placing men at risk? Dare we inquire why our movies, our theater, and even our music portray the gentleman gambler? Dare we wonder, "Does life follow art or does art merely imitate life?"

1. Castellani B., "Is Pathological Gambling Really a Problem?—You bet!" Psychiatric Times, 2001:64

223.   **D**   **All of the above**

Persistent gambling
Recurrent gambling
Maladaptive gambling

Persistent, recurrent, and maladaptive gambling leads to emotional problems, and unemployment. Gambling becomes a coping mechanism albeit a dysfunctional coping mechanism. Our folk mythology of the strong silent man dictates that a man "must" always have resources to cope with any emotional issues and any unemployment and/or underemployment issues. Rather than ask for help or assistance, our strong silent man may simply place bet after bet in a hope to "get lucky" and "win it all back again!"

1. Castellani B., "Is Pathological Gambling Really a Problem?—You bet!" Psychiatric Times, 2001:66.

224.   **E**   **All of the above**

Divorce
Job loss
Financial problems
Strained relationships

These negative consequences lead to emotional distress and legal troubles. Pathological gamblers must deal with not only their impulsivity which started them gambling in the first place but also with multiple losses. There may well appear to be no light at the end of the tunnel of gambling. No matter how much he loses, the pathological gambler is and remains convinced that just one more bet, just one more roll of the dice, will restore his wealth, his health, and his happiness.

1. Castellani B., "Is Pathological Gambling Really a Problem? —You bet!" Psychiatric Times, 2001:66

225.   **B**   **Steadily deteriorate**

Tom's life is expected to steadily deteriorate in a steadily downward spiral:

1. Tom may never have money; or, more properly, Tom may never have enough money.
2. Tom will always dress well, nice suit, white shirt, silk red tie, well spoken, appearing on the surface to be the much the same as anyone else.
3. Tom will always appear to be "flush," or "in the pink;" always "flashing cash," always ready to buy another round of drinks for his gambling buddies or potential gambling buddies.
4. And yet, Tom will always be, "waiting for his ships to come in!"

1. Castellani B., "Is Pathological Gambling Really a Problem? —You bet!" Psychiatric Times, 2001:66.

226.   **B**   **No**

Charles' ongoing alcohol abuse will render an evaluation for dementia null and void. Charles will need to "dry out," and eat a good diet probably with vitamin supplements for an extended period of time prior to any evaluation for dementia. While it is true that Alzheimer's dementia is the most common neurodegenerative in the United States (with Parkinson's Disorder being the second most common neurodegenerative disorder in the United States) the healthcare provider needs to be careful to avoid making the diagnosis of dementia prematurely. The time taken for Charles to "dry out" and to eat a good diet will be rewarded if Charles' sensorium clears following his period of detoxification.

1. Corey-Blum, Jody Audio-Digest Internal Medicine, "Everyday Neurology: Stroke/Cognitive Impairment: Dementia, Delirium, and Memory Loss" Volume 43, Number 10, (Supplement) 1996:4

     Medtext Medical World, Inc.

227.   **E**   25%

In the absence of a transient ischemic attack (T.I.A.), in patients 70 years of age, the risk of stroke may well be 1% per year over a five year period. However, in the presence of a transient ischemic attack (T.I.A) the risk of stroke does not level off for four years and the risk of stroke may well be 25% at 18 months following a transient ischemic attack (T.I.A.)

1. Samuels, M., Audio-Digest Internal Medicine, "Everyday Neurology: Stroke/Cognitive Impairment: Stroke and Cardiovascular Disease," Volume 43, Number 10, (Supplement) 1996:1

228.   **E**   **All of the above**

    Orientation
    Recent and remote memory
    Language
    Apraxia (Inability to perform complex motor acts)

Mental status also includes the perception of visuospatial relations, the ability perform calculations and perhaps the most vital; i.e., judgment.

1. Education may affect the Mini-Mental-Status testing score.

2. Age may affect the Mini-Mental-Status score.

Healthcare provider may choose to obtain repeated Mini-Mental-Status testing over an extending period of time.

1. Corey-Blum, Jody Audio-Digest Internal Medicine, "Everyday Neurology: Stroke/Cognitive Impairment: Dementia, Delirium, and Memory Loss" Volume 43, Number 10. (Supplement) 1996:4.

2. Samuels, M. Audio-Digest Internal Medicine, "Everyday Neurology: Stroke/Cognitive Impairment: Stroke and Cardiovascular Disease," Volume 43, Number 10, (Supplement) 1996:1.

229.   E   50-80%

Alzheimer's Disorder is the most common neurodegenerative disorder in the United States. The initial early phase characterized by the inability to make new memories and visuospatial deficiencies render the individual unable to drive a vehicle is followed by difficulty in comprehension and agitation which may well be associated with a reduction in the ability to cope with the basic activities of daily living which may well include dressing and undressing, keeping clean, and attending to the wants of nature.

1. Corey-Blum, Jody Audio-Digest Internal Medicine, "Everyday Neurology: Stroke/Cognitive Impairment: Dementia, Delirium, and Memory Loss" Volume 43, Number 10, (Supplement) 1996:4

230.   B   Mary

In additional to family history and head trauma, female sex, advanced age and lack of education may well be risk factors for Alzheimer's Disorder.

1. The issue of age is generally accepted in our general patient population.
2. The issue of education is not!

Long term follow up of individuals with varying levels of education in general and variation in the study of multiple languages in particular appeared to reveal that those who studied multiple languages appeared to be at somewhat lower risk of the development of Alzheimer's Disorder.

1. Corey-Blum, Jody Audio-Digest Internal Medicine, "Everyday Neurology: Stroke/Cognitive Impairment: Dementia, Delirium, and Memory Loss" Volume 43, Number 10, (Supplement) 1996:4

231.   **A**   **Capgras' Syndrome**

Capgras' Syndrome (familiar people believed to be impostors) is seen in the intermediate state of Alzheimer's Disorder in association with delusions and paranoia. Encephalotrigeminal Syndrome is manifestation of Sturgi-Weber Disorder characterized by the facial port wine stain, seizures and reduced intellectual functioning; and, Horner's Syndrome is the ptosis, meiosis, enopthalmos, and anhydrosis seen in disorders involving the stellate ganglion.

1. Corey-Blum, Jody Audio-Digest Internal Medicine, "Everyday Neurology: Stroke/Cognitive Impairment: Dementia, Delirium, and Memory Loss" Volume 43, Number 10, (Supplement) 1996:4

232.   **D**   **All of the above**

      Avoidance
      Numbness
      Hyper arousal

In the San Diego Widowhood Project, 350 subjects scored on symptoms of avoidance, numbness and hyper arousal;

1. 10% met the criteria for P.T.S.D. at two months
2. 8% met the criteria for P.T.S.D. at thirteen months
3. 7% met the criteria for P.T.S.D. at two years

The old belief that an expected death was somewhat or somehow easier on the surviving spouse would now appear to be untrue. The old belief that after a period of a few weeks or a few months at most of grieving that the surviving spouse would somehow "get over it," is untrue. We are now in a position to begin to grasp the long term suffering manifested by psychiatric illness of the bereaved.

1. Zisook, S, Audio-Digest Psychiatry "P.T.S.D. After Loss: Bereavement," Volume 29, Issue 12, (Supplement), 2000:1

233.   B   No

In the San Diego Widowhood Project, whether the loss was sudden or expected was irrelevant to the risk of the widow (widower) for Post Traumatic Stress Disorder. The old belief that an expected death was somewhat or somehow easier on the surviving spouse would now appear to be untrue. The old belief that after a period of a few weeks or a few months at most of grieving that the surviving spouse would somehow "get over it," is untrue. We may well be now in a position to begin to grasp the long term suffering manifested by psychiatric illness of the bereaved. These newer or relatively new observations may well be somewhat counterintuitive but are nonetheless true. Facing them may well be a first step in providing a reasonably high quality of psychiatric treatment and care for the bereaved.

1. Zisook, S, Audio-Digest Psychiatry "P.T.S.D. After Loss: Bereavement" Volume 29, Issue 12, (Supplement), 2000:1

234.   D   36%

In the San Diego Widowhood Project, loss of a loved one by accident or suicide had a 36% probability of Post Traumatic Stress Disorder. This figure approximates the probability of Post Traumatic Stress Disorder seen in combat veterans. Healthcare providers can take what has been learned from the treatment and care of the P.T.S.D. of combat veterans and apply it, kindly and gently, to the treatment and care of the P.T.S.D. of the bereaved.

1. Zisook, S, Audio-Digest Psychiatry "P.T.S.D. After Loss: Bereavement" Volume 29, Issue 12, (Supplement), 2000:1

235.   D   Could well be a chronic illness for years

In the San Diego Widowhood Project, the Post Traumatic Stress Disorder tends to be chronic. Of those widows (or widowers) meeting the criteria for P.T.S.D. at two months, 40% met the criteria at one year; and, of those widows (or widowers) meeting the criteria for P.T.S.D. at 1 year, 60% met the criteria for P.T.S.D. at 2 years. Those widows (or widowers) meeting the criteria for P.T.S.D. were less likely to be in a relationship, had poorer relationships with their children, were not working well, and were in suboptimal health.

1. Zisook, S, Audio-Digest Psychiatry "P.T.S.D. After Loss: Bereavement" Volume 29, Issue 12, (Supplement), 2000:1.

236.   C   Tom

Obsessive-Compulsive Disorder (O.C.D.) is a chronic illness waxing and waning in severity. The typical O.C.D patient experiences the onset of O.C.D. at age 13 years; and, is initially seen in a Mental Health Clinic at age 24 years. Healthcare providers and their patients suffering with O.C.D. may well need to lower their expectations somewhat in order to set reasonable goals in therapy. For example, a patient may present with a history of hand washing 75 times a day. For that patient suffering with O.C.D., the reduction of hand washing to 20 times a day may well represent a gain in therapy.

1. Greist, J. Audio-Digest Psychiatry, "Treating Obsessive-Compulsive Disorder," Volume 29, Issue 11, (Supplement) 2000:1.

Medtext Medical World, Inc.

237.   **E**   **None of the above**

Rorschach ink blot tests on Nazi war criminals failed to reveal the presence of any specific mental illness. This observation may well appear to be somewhat counterintuitive (against common-sense). We might anticipate that the atrocities committed in the World War II, European Death Camps including Auschwitz, Bergen Belsen and Dachau might well have been engendered by psychopathology. Such was not the case. Rorschach ink blot testing on these Nazi war criminals revealed no evidence of significant psychopathology.

1. Zillmer E.A., Harrover M., Ritzler B.A., "The Quest for the Nazi Personality: A Psychological Investigation of Nazi War Criminals," Hillsdale, New Jersey, Lawrence Earlbaum Associates. 1995 PAGE #

2. Novac A., "Traumatic Stress and Human Behavior," Psychiatric Times, XVIII, Number 04. 2001:42

238.   **C**   **Trigeminal neuralgia**

Her dental x-rays would have excluded both an impacted wisdom tooth and a jaw abscess. The "jaw aching" of an acute anterior wall myocardial infarction would not be a reasonable consideration in this young, physically fit, non-smoking woman; that is, she has minimal risk factors for the development of an acute myocardial infarction (acute coronary syndrome). Tic Douloureux (Trigeminal neuralgia) is her most reasonable diagnostic consideration.

1. Nathan M.P.R., "A Most Unusual Case," Cortlandt Forum, 2001:66

239.   **C**   **Carbamazepine (Tegretol)**

Haloperidol (Haldol) may be provided for an acute psychosis. Diazepam (Valium) may be provided for alcohol withdrawal. Digoxin (Lanoxin) may be provided to slow the rapid ventricular response to atrial fibrillation. Metformin (Glucophage) may be provided to control the blood glucose level of diabetes mellitus. Carbamazepine (Tegretol) may be expected to relieve partially the pain of her Tic Douloureux (Trigeminal neuralgia).

1. Nathan M.P.R., "A Most Unusual Case," Cortlandt Forum, 2001:66

Medtext Medical World, Inc.

240.   **C**   **Ramsey-Hunt Disorder**

Osler-Weber-Rendu Disorder is hereditary hemorrhagic telangiectatica disorder presenting with an iron deficiency blood loss anemia due to slow and chronic gut bleeds due to internal telangiectasia (tiny bleeding spider-like arterial blood vessels) in the gut associated with telangiectasia of the skin and of the mucous membranes (mouth, lips). Sturge-Weber-Dimiti Disorder is the encephalotrigeminal syndrome presenting with a facial port wine strain (birthmark), on the face in the distribution of the trigeminal (5th cranial) nerve presenting with reduced intellectual functioning and generalized seizures. Our patient, "Bill," has the Ramsey-Hunt Disorder presenting with a facial paralysis due to a viral involvement of the dorsal-root ganglion of his facial (7th cranial) nerve.

1. Glatt A.E., "A Most Unusual Case," Cortlandt Forum, 2001:67

241.   **A**   **Varicella (chickenpox virus)**

Spousal abuse (husband abuse) is an unreasonable consideration as wives rarely abuse their husbands. While malignant cells can invade the mental branch of the trigeminal (5th) cranial nerve and can, rarely, present with a "numb chin" syndrome, malignancy would not be the first and most probable consideration in this otherwise young healthy father of otherwise healthy young children. Perhaps the best proof of Varicella viral involvement of Bill's dorsal root ganglion of his facial (7th cranial) nerve was that his daughter developed chickenpox (another Varicella manifestation) in two weeks.

1. Glatt A.E., "A Most Unusual Case," Cortlandt Forum, 2001:67

242.   **D**   **Acyclovir**

Zidovudine, Lamivudine, Indinavir, have been used in combination for highly active anti-retroviral (H.A.A.R.T.) pharmacotherapy in patients with the Acquired Immune Deficiency Syndrome (A.I.D.S.). These and the non-steroidal pharmaceuticals such as ibuprofen (Motrin) have no reasonable place in the treatment of a dorsal-root ganglion Varicella involvement. Acyclovir (high-dose, oral) is the reasonable treatment of choice.

1. Glatt A.E., "A Most Unusual Case," Cortlandt Forum, 2001:67

243.   **E**   **All of the above**

         Neck pain
         Headache
         Photophobia
         Paresthesias in the right arm

Sandra's neck pain, headache, and photophobia (sensitivity of the eyes to light such that bright light actually causes pain and bright light is avoided by the patient) are to be reasonably expected in this instance of head trauma. Perhaps the most significant, of those listed, may well be her localizing finding of paresthesias in her right arm associated with the weakness of her right arm.

1. Brown, M.F., "Carotid Artery Injuries," American Journal of Surgery," 1982; 144:748

Medtext Medical World, Inc.

244.   E   Traumatic Carotid Artery Dissection

Sandra initially was a vibrant, healthy young woman. Prior to her bike-wreck she was employed full time and was in a relationship albeit a somewhat emotionally abusive relationship. Therefore we would not diagnose brain tumor, brain abscess, amyotrophic lateral sclerosis (A.L.S.), or multiple sclerosis (M.S.) in the absence of chronic pre-trauma signs and symptoms. The impact of Sandra's jaw on the concrete associated with the localizing findings of weakness and paresthesias of Sandra's right arm brings a traumatic carotid-artery dissection into reasonable consideration. The most significant portion of the neurological examination is the presence of localizing or lateralizing neurologic signs and symptoms that point directly to her carotid artery trauma.

1. Loscalzo, J., Creager, M.A., and Dzau, V.J., (Editors) "Blunt Vascular Trauma in Vascular Medicine," First Edition, Little, Brown, and Company, 1992: 1158

245.   A   III

Paralysis of the sixth (6th) cranial nerve (abducens) will lead to failure of abduction of the extra-ocular muscles. The first (1st) cranial nerve (olfactory) provides the sense of smell. The fifth (5th) cranial nerve (trigeminal) provides sensation of the face and cornea. The seventh (7th) cranial nerve (facial) provides muscular movement of the face. A branch of Sandra's third (3rd) cranial nerve (occulomotor nerve) can be affected by her traumatic carotid artery dissection thus producing Sandra's anisocoria (unequal pupils). Sandra's new-onset anisocoria (unequal pupils) is a localizing and lateralizing neurologic sign which points directly to her carotid artery trauma.

1. Adams, R.D and Victor M., (Editors), "Cranial Nerve Syndromes in Principles of Neurology," Fifth Edition, McGraw-Hill, Incorporated, Health Professions Division, 1993: 1173

246. **Patients receiving workers compensation payments for pain are considered to be at two to three times greater risk for suicide than the general population**

Although there is a dearth of data on the subject of suicide completion within the chronic pain population, it is generally felt that this group is at significant risk. Caucasian men and women, aged 35 to 64 years, receiving workers' compensation for pain, were shown to be at two to three times greater risk for suicide than the general population. This rate was however significantly lower than that seen in a psychiatric population. Despite this one study's limitations, the authors concluded that chronic pain patients are at significant risk for suicide.

1. Fishbain, D.A., Goldberg, M., Rosomoff, R. S., Rosomoff, H: Completed suicide in chronic pain. Clin J Pain 7(2):29-36, 1991.

247. **B** **About one third of individuals reporting headaches and related pain complaints following a motor vehicle accident meet the criteria for post traumatic stress disorder**

Symptoms of post traumatic stress disorder may commonly follow motor vehicles accidents, work-related injuries, or violent crime. Pain is a common concomitant of the disorder. Significant impairment of functioning is an essential clinical feature of post traumatic stress disorder in the DSM-IV. Systematic desensitization is a behavioral technique that has been shown to be quite successful treating phobias and has been successfully applied to pain patients with post traumatic stress disorder. Psychological trauma often goes unnoticed by medical professionals who are often focused on the medical physical aspects of the patient following accidents and injuries. Delays in functional recovery are often related to psychological trauma.

1. Muse, M., Stress-related, post-traumatic chronic pain syndrome: Behavioral treatment approach. Pain 25(3):389-394, 1986

Medtext Medical World, Inc.

248.　　　E　　NSAIDS are associated with hyperkalemia

Although nausea and vomiting can be produced by NSAIDS, dyspepsia is in fact a poor predictor for NSAID induced ulceration or perforation. NSAIDS can cause hyponatremia and hyperkalemia as a result of altered renal function. In addition, the action of antidiuretic hormone may be increased, exacerbating congestive heart failure and raising lithium levels. An analgesic should not be considered a failure unless it has been pushed to the maximum tolerated dose. For benign pain conditions, 2 weeks of a maximal dose constitute an adequate trial. For malignant pain conditions, 1 week is considered sufficient.

1. Portenoy, R. K.: Principles of treatment with nonopioid analgesics and adjuvant drugs: Post graduate course. In Current Concepts in Acute, Chronic and Cancer Pain Management, 1993.

249.　　　A　　Buprenorphine

When a drug combines with a receptor site to produce the action of the receptor it is considered an agonist. A drug that binds with a receptor and inhibits activity is considered an antagonist. Semi-synthetic and synthetic products have been produced that are both agonist and antagonist. The hope in producing these drugs was that they would be agonist for analgesic affects and antagonist for the respiratory depression and sedative effects of the opioids. Examples of common mixed agonist-antagonist opioid drugs include: butorphanol, buprenorphine, and pentazocine. The other drugs listed are agonists.

1. Porter, J., Jick, H.: Addiction rare in patients treated with narcotics. N Engl J Med 302:123, 1980.

250.   **C**   **Methadone**

Of the drugs listed, methadone has the longest serum half-life which makes methadone a useful drug for opiate detoxification. The other medications listed all have short serum half-lives.   Although fentanyl has a short serum half-life, the delivery system for transdermal fentanyl is designed to allow the patch to be changes every 48 to 72 hours. Methadone is available in both oral and intra-muscular routes.   Buprenorphine is now available for outpatient office based opiate detoxification. The opportunity to detox from opiates away from the methadone clinic environment may offer specific clinical advantages for many patients.

1. Porter, J., Jick, H.: Addiction rare in patients treated with narcotics. N Engl J Med 302:123, 1980.

Medtext Medical World, Inc.

Good Luck!

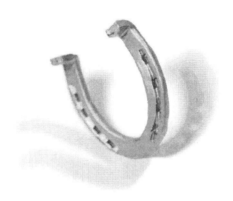

From Medtext

Let us know your test results! We love hearing from our customers.
Send a message to info@medtext.net